MW01108459

See pp. 12-13; 103-107

A Woman Ahead Of Her Time

Praise for
A Woman Ahead Of Her Time

Anne Evans has given us an engaging and loving account of one remarkable woman, ahead of her time even as a young woman. Maida
Solomon's journey, chronicled in personal letters, diary entries, and
jottings, is inspiring testimony to the social rewards of one person's dedication and commitment to humanitarian instincts. With this memoir,
both Evans and Solomon have enriched our social awareness.

Don R. Lipsitt, MD
Chairman Emeritus, Department of Psychiatry
Mt. Auburn Hospital, Cambridge, MA

Professor of Psychiatry, Harvard Medical School

Editor in Chief, *General Hospital Psychiatry*

★ ★ ★

Anne Evans has done a masterful job of bringing Maida Herman Solomon and her achievements to life for all of us to admire and enjoy. *A
Woman Ahead of Her Time* vividly portrays a woman, born in 1891, who
challenged the existing social structure of the early 1900s and forged
ahead to become a 20th-century leader in developing and teaching psychiatric social work. She was a model and an inspiration for young
women in the integration of work, wife and mother roles.

Maida Solomon's personal life comes alive in excerpts from her diaries and letters, while her remarkable professional achievements are
documented through statements that accompanied presentations of
awards. Her early years at home are briefly described, followed by discussion of her rapid personal and intellectual growth and independence
in college. Her years of work are described beautifully. Especially
meaningful are accounts of her personal qualities and beliefs, which ac-

counted for her leadership role in the development of psychiatric social work and the place of women in our society.

After mandatory retirement from teaching at the Simmons College School of Social Work, Maida Solomon went on to a career in research and to mentoring young professional women. This period is richly informed by oral history accounts.

Carolyn B. Thomas, PhD
Professor Emeritus, Boston College School of Social Work, Boston, MA

★ ★ ★

This is a story about a life well lived, and it is a story well told. Maida Herman Solomon's remarkable life spanned a significant part of the twentieth century with themes of fundamental possibilities and transformation for women and for the field of social work.

Anne Evans, combining her own sense of professional commitment, her affection for a most valued teacher, and her skill in story telling, shows us this world with exuberant tenderness. She succeeds in providing us with the experiential immediacy necessary for feeling, imagining, and knowing what it was like for Maida Solomon to meet the enormous challenges of those days with energy, pioneer spirit, and professional dedication.

Today, in our complex world, with still enormous, yet difficult challenges before us, we must continue to honor the legacy of those who came before and gave us the foundations to build upon and move forward.

Anne Evans' biography of Maida Solomon is a welcome addition to our social work collection. It is a book that will serve as a valuable source of information and inspiration for all social workers for many years to come.

Golnar S. Simpson, DSW, BCD
Chair, National Academy of Practice in Social Work

Past President, Clinical Social Work Federation

Founding Dean, Clinical Social Work Institute, Washington, DC

The biography of Maida Herman Solomon (1891–1996) chronicles her life and extraordinary career as one of a very small group of colleagues who created, nurtured, and developed the profession of psychiatric social work. Her earliest research with her husband, Dr. Harry Caesar Solomon, at the Boston Psychopathic Hospital culminated with the publication of the classic book *Syphilis of the Innocent* in 1920.

Her career moved from the psychiatric hospital to the Massachusetts Department of Social Hygiene prior to her being invited to join the faculty at Simmons College in 1934. There she was given the mandate to develop a two-year graduate program in Psychiatric Social Work. After her mandatory retirement in 1957, Mrs. Solomon was invited to return to the Boston Psychopathic Hospital to fill the newly created position of Consultant in Social Psychiatry and Social Work Research. She consulted to many of her former students in a variety of settings into her nineties.

As a friend and a colleague of Maida and Harry Solomon, Mrs. Evans had unusual access to diaries, interviews with colleagues, and personal recollections of Solomon family members. She has used her source materials effectively to capture the essence of a remarkable personality. So, too, Dr. Miles Shore's introduction recounts in lively detail his experiences of "Mrs. S." Particularly touching is the eulogy given by Rabbi H. Bruce Ehrmann at her private memorial service.

Mary T. Breslin, MSW

A Woman Ahead Of Her Time
Maida Herman Solomon,
Mental Health Visionary

Anne Sugarman Evans, MSW
Introduction by Miles F. Shore, MD

Many thanks for allowing me to reprint your brief eulogy. It has added a personal insight that could not have been duplicated elsewhere.

Anne Evans

September 2003

Coastal Villages Press
Beaufort, South Carolina

Tabby Manse

Published by Coastal Villages Press,
a division of Coastal Villages, Inc.,
PO Box 6300, Beaufort, SC 29903,
843-524-0075, fax 843-525-0000,
a publisher of books since 1992.
Visit our web site: www.coastal-villages.com.

Available at special discounts for bulk purchases
and sales promotions from the publisher
and your local bookseller.

Cover illustration by Nona Rooney.
Photographs by permission of
Schlesinger Library, Radcliffe Institute, Harvard University;
The Simmons College Archives;
Mr. & Mrs. Joseph Herman Solomon;
and Dr. Edward Sugarman.

ISBN 1-882943-19-8
Library of Congress Control Number: 2003110317

First Edition
Printed in the United States of America

To MHS,
teacher, mentor, colleague, friend,
and to my family

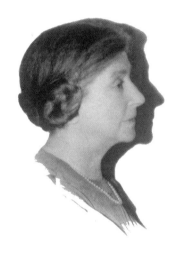

Contents

Preface

Maida Herman Solomon (1891-1988) has been recognized as a pioneer among a very small group of social work professionals who "invented" the field of psychiatric social work. She oversaw its definition, its development of standards, and its integration with the other institutions of modern American medicine and education. She helped found the profession of psychiatric social work.

So too, she developed a curricula that moved social work at the Simmons College School of Social Work, Boston, MA, from an undergraduate program to a two-year graduate Master of Social Work (MSW) professional degree.

Upon her retirement from Simmons in 1957, at age sixty-six, she returned to the Massachusetts Mental Health Center (formerly Boston Psychopathic Hospital) as a consultant in social psychiatry and social work research. In this role, in which she worked into her early nineties, she helped many young professional social workers combine their careers with marriage and children, thus transplanting her own belief system to those of her young colleagues.[1]

The portrait of this remarkable woman within her family, among her friends, and throughout her career as a mental health innovator from 1915 onward, requires some knowledge of this historical period and her role as a woman. The reader of this biography will gain a greater understanding of the period by reading a work by Dorothy and Carl J. Schneider entitled *American Women in the Progressive Era, 1900-1920.*[2]

The many-faceted personality of Maida Solomon becomes evident from the remarks of friends, colleagues, and offspring. At age ninety-six, with four children and their spouses, twelve grandchildren, and eleven great-grandchildren[3], she had about her the appearance of a wise matriarch. Comments show her to have been serious, literate, and frank, but with a sense of fun. She was pragmatic in nature with a strong professional identity, and endlessly loyal in her relationships. With students and colleagues, she expected excellence and precision.

Not to be minimized was her stance as a role model for women in the way she combined her work with her role as wife and mother. Maida's attitude flew in the face of college-educated women of her generation who felt they had to make a choice between marriage and a career.[4] As a result, she made it possible for her students, and later her social work colleagues, to integrate their career ambitions with family by advocating a part-time program at Simmons, as well as part-time social work research programs in the mental hospital setting. She often argued that research grant money was far better spent on part-time workers, as they would often give more time proportionately to their work than would a full-time employee.

Maida Herman Solomon was one who, throughout her life, constantly sought challenges. In 1957, at sixty-six years of age, after "retiring" for only a few days as Professor of Social Economy at the Simmons College School of Social Work (recently renamed the Simmons Graduate School of Social Work), she became a consultant in social psychiatry to the Boston Psychopathic Hospital.

Her enthusiasm for her work was enormous. As a result of an advertising campaign for the Volunteer Case Aide Program at the Boston State Hospital, Maida Solomon was among the first to put a bumper sticker on her car that read, "Loneliness Kills."[5]

Her honesty was most telling when she was asked if she was a graduate of a school of social work. She would acknowledge that she was not. Ironically, she was one of a small group who had written the very first curriculum and its qualifying exams, but never matriculated through the two-year Master of Social Work program.

Maida Herman Solomon herself expressed satisfaction with the life she had lived. In anticipation of death, she wrote in a note to her son Joe, "We've had a great time together on earth, with all our kids, their spouses, their kids and their spouses."

At Maida Herman Solomon's private memorial service in 1988, Rabbi H. Bruce Ehrmann stated that "perhaps it was the evident dispar-

Preface

ity between her own favored situation and the problem[5] borne by so much of humanity that prompted her to devote her energies in such large measure to the welfare of fellow people."

Anne S. Evans

July 2003

Notes to Preface

1 Hyman, Paula E. and Moore, Deborah Dash, (ed.), *Jewish Women in America: An Historical Encyclopedia,* 1997, Vol. 2, p.1287.
2 Schneider, Dorothy, and Schneider, Carl J., *American Women in the Progressive Era: 1900-1920,* Doubleday, New York, 1979. See especially pp. 74-76 and 79-80.
3 Family Tree, prepared by David Solomon.
4 Solomon, Barbara Miller, *In the Company of Educated Women: A History of Women in Higher Education in America,* 1985, p. 118.
5 Bumper stickers were one means to recruit volunteers into the Boston State Hospital; Case Aide Program, Boston, MA.

Introduction

One afternoon in the late fall of 1981, I called on Harry and Maida Solomon at their ample Victorian house on a shady street in the Jamaica Plain section of Boston. I was then the superintendent of the Massachusetts Mental Health Center, the job that Harry held from 1943 to 1959. Once or twice a year I would check in with him about the latest events, and ask his advice about what to do. It was unusually warm for the season and I was not surprised to hear the thunk of tennis balls coming from the tennis court out of sight behind the house. I rang the doorbell and after a considerable delay, Maida appeared at the door in her tennis dress. She apologized profusely for making me wait. "I was out in back practicing my serve. It hasn't been very good lately, and I asked Harry to watch out the window while I did a hundred serves. He said I was getting better."

I was in no way surprised at her way of spending the afternoon in what was likely her 90th year. For I had been aware of her formidable spirit ever since I was a psychiatric trainee in the mid-1950s at what was then the Boston Psychopathic Hospital. My initial acquaintance with her was largely "below the stairs," as befitted a first-year resident. That distance, however, gave me a perspective on her stature that could not have been the same had I been closer to the senior levels of the hospital. It was clear to me that she was a powerful force both in the hospital and in the larger world of mental health. I came to that conclusion because she was followed around the hospital by a devoted multidisciplinary coterie of investigators who, I eventually learned, explored professional domains that were far ahead of the fashion of the time.

That was early in the era when an unprecedented number of bright medical school graduates chose to enter psychiatric training, attracted by the lure of psychoanalytic theory and practice. Even at the Boston Psychopathic Hospital, whose defining characteristic was treating seriously ill patients with schizophrenia and other major mental disorders, psychoanalytic treatment had the highest status, and other forms of treatment were regarded as distinctly second-class.

In that atmosphere of rancorous unorthodoxy, Maida Solomon found a congenial welcome for her work on topics outside the mainstream. A full twenty years before managed care provided financial imperatives, she explored ways to prevent hospitalization. For many in psychiatry, the hospital was the place for definitive treatment of mental disorders. Based on the idea that it was possible to work through the psychological conflicts that were supposed to be the root cause of serious mental illnesses, hospitalization for long periods was considered the premier way of curing serious mental disorders even in the mid-1950s, the early days of psychopharmacology.

Maida Solomon and her colleagues saw it differently. For them, it was better to prevent hospitalization, itself a regressive experience. Taking people off the waiting list for admission to the hospital, she and her social work colleagues developed alternatives to hospitalization. It would be a number of years before other investigators validated the notion that short hospital stays based on psychopharmacology were at least as good as, and sometimes better than, long stays. The revolution of community treatment that built on these studies, and a belief of normalization of experience, provided further proof that her ideas were in the vanguard of progress. More recently, of course, the resource limitations that have resulted in managed care have reinforced the importance of finding alternatives to in-patient care.

The idea that acute psychosis resulted from a failure of psychological defenses, melted down by intolerable emotional conflicts, assumed that patients were vulnerable because of defective ways of coping with reality. These personality defects were felt to be the product of bad parenting in the early years. The "schizophrenogenic mother" was an indictment cloaked in psychiatric jargon that convinced therapists to ostracize family members with thinly veiled contempt, and added a burden of intimidation to persons who were already laden with the sadness of lost dreams for their afflicted children.

Introduction

Rather than following the clinical fashion that emphasized patients' weaknesses and defects, Maida Solomon focused on assets that could be enhanced and expanded to assist patients to be successful in their lives. In doing so, she was laying the groundwork through social work for the growing discipline of psychiatric rehabilitation, which sought successful functioning as the goal of treatment. Psychiatric rehabilitation, with its emphasis on patient strengths, is arguably the conceptual basis for the most important modern advances in the care of patients with serious mental disorders. It has spawned social clubs and social-vocational rehabilitation programs, and supported group homes and other residential facilities, all of which serve to normalize the environment for persons with serious disorders. Along with better medications and biological theories of serious mental disorders, these ideas have brought patients with serious disorders back into the mainstream of humanity, helping to reduce the stigmatization of mental illness. These new attitudes have helped to exonerate parents of total responsibility for ruining their children's lives. Family members, no longer relegated by guilt to the closet, have emerged and created the National Alliance for the Mentally Ill (NAMI), perhaps the most effective health-related advocacy group in the country. NAMI has been a potent political force, supporting psychiatric research and improved funding for treatment. And it has provided enormous assistance to families by providing a network of peer support groups. Indeed, Maida Solomon's work in psychiatric rehabilitation facilitated this fundamental change in the way serious mental illnesses are viewed by professionals and by the public.

But of course, her career at the Boston Psychopathic Hospital (shortly to become the Massachusetts Mental Health Center) was only the most recent episode in a life of breaking new ground—although those of us who were new to the field were unaware of her earlier professional incarnations. We were, however, aware of her unusual status as a highly regarded woman academic. And we also observed her vital relationship with her husband.

Like other hospitals founded in the early years of the twentieth century, the Massachusetts Mental Health Center had originally welcomed a significant number of women to its medical staff. In the early years, Dr. Anna Wellington, Chief of the Outpatient Department, and Dr. Myrtelle Canavan, who directed Dr. E. E. Southard's neuro-pathology laboratory, and psychiatric house officers like Dr. Luella Cole, played significant roles in the hospital. And, of course, from the earliest days of the hospital, Maida Solomon was actively involved as a research social worker in the Division of Research on Brain Syphilis, headed by her husband. A photograph from that period shows her with Dr. Southard, the first director, and Harry Solomon in the office of the Division, hard at work at their desks. She is a strikingly beautiful young woman, unself-consciously stylish in high button shoes and a skirt trimmed in fur, conveying her intensity and seriousness of purpose.

By the 1950s, the Boston Psychopathic Hospital, like other medical institutions, was just beginning to experience the re-entry of women into medicine and academic pursuits. This followed a lean period in the late 1920s and 1930s when women had been squeezed out of academic and professional medical careers. Women physicians, grudgingly admitted to medical training during World War II when male applicants were scarce, were reaching the first stages of professional maturity. And medical schools, with Harvard slowly catching up with the trends, were beginning to admit more women. Psychiatric social workers, like young physicians, were interested in psychoanalytic psychotherapy, and training in that field was expanding. But there were few women who were mature academic investigators. Preeminent among these was Maida Solomon, a role model for women with professional interests and aspirations, and a lesson for men who had the opportunity to learn how to relate to a woman of professional stature.

There was another lesson for all of us, both men and women, to be found in the relationship between Maida Solomon and her husband. The two-career marriage was in its infancy, but the Massachusetts Mental Health Center offered two examples. Milton Greenblatt was the assistant superintendent, and a central figure as research director; his wife, Gertrude Rogers, was a child psychiatrist and the director of the in-patient service for children. But the most high-profile two-career couple was the Solomons. Their first professional collaboration on the syphilis project had been interrupted by her appointment in 1934 as Professor of Social Economy and head of the psychiatric social work program at Simmons College School of Social Work. Upon her retirement from Simmons, in 1957, Harry Solomon called up Milton Greenblatt; "Maida is restless," he said. "Can you find something for her to do?" With characteristic gusto, Greenblatt found her three jobs immediately, giving her the title of Consultant in Psychiatric Social Work Research. From the vantage point of a psychiatric resident, it was enlightening to see how they were both separate and apart. They were like championship ice dancers who coordinated their moves, always in the same arena, but apart as often as together. Yet again, Maida Solomon was ahead of her time.

For more than seventy years, beginning in 1914, she worked to define psychiatric social work (now described as clinical social work) as a profession which she envisioned as having a vital and distinctive place in mental health practice. As Jill K. Conway, President of Smith College, said in presenting the prestigious Smith College Medal to Maida, "To recount the significant points in your career is to describe the establishment of your profession."

Living well into one's tenth decade may or may not be a blessing. At the very least it gives scope for one's influence for better or worse, to be spread across the canvas of time. Maida Solomon made extraordinary use of the unusual amount of time that she was granted. Her influence as a pioneer in psychiatric social work, in social work research, and in laying the empirical and intellectual groundwork for significant developments in the treatment of mental illnesses would have been enormous had she died many years earlier. That she continued to contribute for so long was an inestimable gift to her and to all of us.

Miles F. Shore, MD
Bullard Professor of Psychiatry,
Harvard Medical School

Visiting Scholar, Kennedy School of Government,
Harvard University, 1999

A Woman Ahead Of Her Time

I
Childhood

Maida Herman, born on March 9, 1891, was the third daughter and last child of Joseph Michael and Hannah (always called Hennie) Adler Herman of Columbus Avenue in Boston, MA. This part of the South End was "just a bit below the upper middle class...not a Jewish neighborhood, but better off German Jews lived on Columbus Avenue and Tremont Street."[1]

Maida described her childhood as "extremely lonely." She was seven years younger than her next sister Babette (Bess) and she remembered that "sometimes they chose to let me tag along with them and other times they didn't." At seven Maida attended the Prince School on Newbury Street, a public school within walking distance of home. "I tagged along with my sister who went to the Latin School. The Prince School was a very gloomy place, and I believe there wasn't room for me in the kindergarten. So I went to first grade right away."[2] During this period, Maida had a "best friend," Martha Eliot, who was ahead of Maida in school. They both graduated from Prince and moved on to the Girls' Latin School, ninth grade (fourth class). There was apparently no entrance exam requirement. Maida was a conscientious student, deciding not to go to the St. Louis World's Fair on a family trip, as she wanted to stay home and "finish my work." As a result, her mother took the two older daughters, Sarah and Bess, and her father remained at home with Maida.

Her parents were members of the Reform Congregation Temple Israel of Boston. Maida refused to go to Sunday school, although both Sarah and Bess attended. "Somehow they couldn't resist as strongly as I."[3] Maida's rebellion was not entirely unfounded in her parent's attitudes.

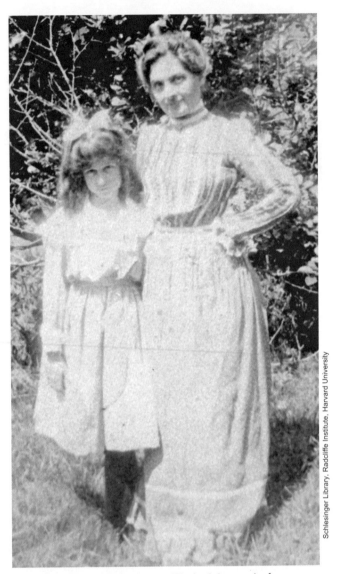

Schlesinger Library, Radcliffe Institute, Harvard University

Maida Herman, age 8, at Twin Mountain house,
New Hampshire, with her German nurse, 1899.

Childhood

Her mother came from a religious family in Baltimore and married Joseph when she was only nineteen. Joseph showed little interest in temple, attending only on the High Holidays at the start of the Jewish New Year.

Early in their marriage, Hennie Herman was "exposed" to Mrs. Lina Hecht, a great-aunt of Maida's who was later a huge influence on Maida as well. Both Mr. and Mrs. Hecht were important philanthropists in Boston; their interests extended throughout the community to both nonsectarian and Jewish causes. Lina Hecht was instrumental in establishing scholarships for needy girls to attend college at Radcliffe. With other affluent Jewish families, including the Hermans, she established the Hebrew Industrial School for Girls, later renamed the Hecht Neighborhood House. The young Mrs. Herman was taken under Aunt Lina's wing and attended religious services with her.

The distinguished business leader and philanthropist Louis Kirstein paid the following tribute to the Hechts at the dedication of the Hecht Neighborhood House on January 19, 1936:

> I leave it to others today to dwell on the present and the future of the institution, which we are dedicating today. I prefer to use my name to pay tribute to the memory of those who had the vision years ago to lay the foundation for the service which the Hecht Neighborhood House symbolizes. I want to talk about Mr. and Mrs. Jacob Hecht, about 'Uncle Jake and Aunt Lina,' as they were affectionately known to those who had the privilege of coming within their circle. Nothing worthwhile is created without vision and without effort. Every worthwhile institution and movement has its history, and behind that history are the understanding and vision of people who begin things. Mr. and Mrs. Jacob Hecht belong to this small group. They had concern for their fellow men of all classes, regardless of economic status, regardless of race or religion.
>
> Aunt Lina's home was, a generation ago, the leading intellectual and spiritual center of the Jewish community of Boston. It was there that students from Harvard and other colleges assembled for social and intellectual intercourse. It was there that distinguished visitors from all over the world came when they visited Boston. There was grace and beauty and nobility in that atmosphere which they created, but they were not

content simply with the influence they might exert within their domestic environment.

Two important community organizations sprang from that home. Mr. Hecht launched one; he was one of the chief founders of the Hebrew Benevolent Association, and, with his brother Louis and Joseph M. Herman [Maida's father] and other good men, did much to raise the social conscience of the Jewish men and women of Boston [so that] immigrants and other underprivileged would be given a helping hand…in their new home.

That Hebrew Benevolent Association laid the foundation for what is now the Associated Jewish Philanthropies [in 1990 renamed the Combined Jewish Philanthropies], one of the leading Jewish federations in the country.

Aunt Lina was a deeply spiritual and religious person. It was her vision that led to the establishment of the Industrial School. She inspired the young Jewish women [among them Hennie Herman, Maida's mother] to help her. From the Industrial School sprang the institution which we are dedicating today, the new Hecht Neighborhood House. [Maida would later serve as a board member.] It became the center of high companionship, a place where rich and poor, the high and lowly, met in equal status, both working for the common good…

And so to those pioneers of another generation, I want to pay my modest tribute today. I want to remember them for my own sake, for when I came as a stranger to the City of Boston, more than fifty years ago, they took me in and made me feel at home. They played their part in shaping my thoughts, and whatever service I may have been able to give to our community, no doubt drew large inspiration from their example…

Let their lives and their deeds be a symbol and reminder to all of us of the opportunities before us for service, if we will but have the vision and the courage. It is fitting that the name 'Hecht' should be engraved in this Institution. It is the kind of immortality which would have pleased Mr. and Mrs. Hecht most.[4]

Undoubtedly this interest in community affairs and philanthropy had a great impact on the young Maida and became indelibly printed on her developing character and persona. Aunt Lina Hecht was indeed a mentor to the impressionable Maida Herman as much as to her mother. "It was with horror that I discovered that I didn't originate good works on my own," she would later say. "I inherited good works."[5]

Childhood

When Maida was ten, the family moved to Marlborough Street in Boston's Back Bay neighborhood. The move brought the family together around the intellectual and social commitments represented by the Hechts. The Hermans lunched every Saturday at the Hechts' large Commonwealth Avenue home. Maida recalled "quantities of silver...and chairs...and food spread over tables." It was in that setting at Saturday lunch that "an attempt was made to give us a mild Jewish education."[6] At the time Maida reported also being "exposed" to Christmas, "which made quite a difference in my general attitude towards life and the upbringing of my children." Her sister's best friend came from Germany, and that family, though Jewish, brought the idea of the Christmas tree with them. Maida loved the tree and chose to have a tree in her own home for many years while her children were growing up.

Perhaps the most significant trauma Maida suffered in her childhood and early adolescence was the diagnosis and treatment of a tubercular gland first noticed when she was two. It set her apart in her own mind and taught her a characteristic kind of strength. She said later:

> First I coped with it by retreat [shyness] when I was little...five, six, seven. But when I got to be nine or ten I said this is it and I will wear my hair this way. When I got to be thirteen [1904], I was exposed to (at that time) modern experimental treatment of glandular disease...I [learned] it could be cancerous...and then I came to realize the affection my father had for me, because he didn't want me to be operated on as he was afraid I would die, so we did this other experimental thing...having X-ray treatments which had not yet been perfected.
>
> I was burned by the X-ray, which increased the cosmetic problem...the medical treatment didn't work of course and...gave me a high temperature and the doctors came...and they punched [lanced] it and I went through a good deal of emotional difficulty and I became then a different kind of person...[more] independent...in my own mind, a brave person who would face life, never mind what happened to me or what anybody else said to me, that was it!
>
> In those days you stayed at home, you didn't go to hospitals...I had an operation in spite of my father's anxiety and it turned out all right. For a year or so I had really bad scars, which I covered, and I said to myself, this is the way you are and the rest of you is rather good looking.[7]

Throughout her life she never laid her troubles at other peoples' feet, but always turned her private problems into strengths others could admire. As photographs of her show, she was, throughout her life, a handsome woman.

While Maida was going through her surgery and recuperation, her older sisters were entering maturity. Sarah was not interested in college, but went to "finishing school" instead, where she took courses in art and music and became quite an accomplished pianist. Bess wanted to attend Smith, but her father would not hear of her going so far away from home. (The trip from Boston to Northampton, in the early 20th century, was a half-day by train and bus.) Instead, Bess went to Radcliffe College (then the Women's College of Harvard University and now the Radcliffe Institute of Harvard University) as a day student, because her father would not allow her to live on campus.

In many ways Maida's sisters led the way for her. She learned much from them, not only from their example, but also from their conversations. Young Maida's sex education, for instance, took place when she was nine or ten. Her nurse got married and Maida noticed that the nurse's body got 'mildly bigger.' "I spoke to my sister who said that maybe I would have things happen to me later. When the nurse's baby came, I accepted it...watched its growth, etc....but other sex information came somewhat premenstrual, when it seemed wise to my sister and me that I should hear more about these things before I started noticing blood or anything."

And she learned too about other matters from her mother. Although Maida had resisted formal religious education, as an older girl she sought her mother's point of view and advice. In one of her early diaries (1905) Maida wrote:

> I asked Mother to come up to my room. She came. At first I was a little weeny embarrassed because I never really talked about the things I did talk about before...then I spoke about religion. I told Mother that I wanted religion and I do, I do. Mother told me religion meant to [be] kind to the poor and to do something to help them; to do right and always keep to the narrow path, that is the path of good, and to be strong in right and not let others lead me astray; to believe in God, that he is a

spirit and that people, when they are dead, do not die but live hereafter, and when a dear one dies, feel that you haven't lost them but that you will meet them [again]…if a murderer escapes, his conscience punishes him. A beautiful idea is to think of God on a judgment seat and everybody comes and receives judgment. Therefore, one should aim to do good.[8]

Shortly before she entered Girls' Latin School, Maida's social life began expanding. In 1903 she and four friends decided to form a club and meet on a regular basis. The officers of this newly formed Pickwick Club[9] included May F. Koshland, president; Helen L. Strauss, vice

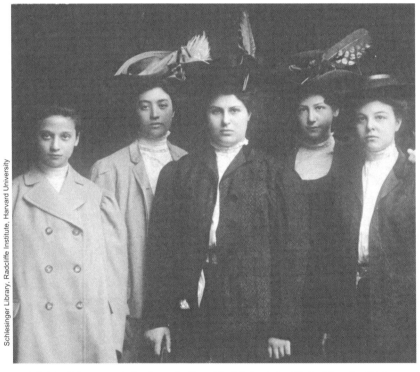

Maida Herman (4th from left) with Pickwick Club friends: Helen Strauss, Fanny Frank, May Koshland, and Ethel Koshland, c. 1907.

president; Fanny Frank, secretary; Maida Herman, treasurer; and Ethel J. Koshland, chairman. An event, presumably for the parents and friends of the members, was held at the Victoria Hotel on Sunday, November 10. Among the offerings in an elegantly printed program was a "Tableaux from Little Women—Mothers and Daughters." The cast included "Marmie," Fannie Frank; "Meg," May F. Koshland; "Jo," Maida Herman; "Beth," Helen L. Strauss; and "Amy," played by Ethel J. Koshland.

Apparently the idea of charity was emphasized as one of the club's missions, as evidenced in the following letter to Mrs. J. M. Herman, Maida's mother, on July 5, 1904:

> Dear Madam:
>   Referring to my last letter, I have much pleasure in handing you certificates; one for each member of the Pickwick Club, in recognition of their thoughtfulness and great kindness in sending us a generous contribution for the Floating Hospital babies. I trust these will remind the members of the club of our gratitude to them and be evidence of our wishes for their happiness and success in all they do for the good of others. The money will help to do a great deal this summer. Although the hospital does not open until tomorrow, for more than a week applications for rooms for sick babies have been coming to us, and we look forward to a busy summer. Personally, I am touched by the evidence of earnest work for the hospital, which this gift gives, and with thanks to you for your kindness in the matter, I am,
>
>   Sincerely,
>   (signed) Rufus B. Tobey, Chairman

As one might assume, the education received at Girls' Latin School was classical and rigorous and included Latin and Greek, as well as history, English, and mathematics. Because languages were "important to the family" (French and German in fact were taught in the home), Maida found Latin School to be quite easy.[10] She graduated in 1908.

In the school yearbook, Jabberwock, a prophetic statement was written beside Maida Herman's name: "If the crowns of all the kingdoms of the empire were laid at her feet in exchange for her books and her love of reading, she would spurn them all."[11]

Childhood

Notes to Chapter 1: Childhood

1 Quoted from Maida Herman Solomon Oral Memoirs, American Jewish Committee, 3 volumes paginated consecutively, 1:000. Subsequent references will appear in the text. Ibid, 1:1
2 ibid., 1:2, 1:3
3 ibid., 1:9
4 Louis Kirstein, address on the occasion of the dedication of the Hecht Neighborhood House, January 19, 1936.
5 ibid., 1:16
6 ibid., 1:12, 1:10
7 ibid., 1:45, 1:47-48
8 from a diary entry, "October 9, 1905, Day of Atonement"
9 In reviewing this section, Eric Solomon, PhD, (Maida and Harry's youngest son) wrote: "All enamored of Charles Dickens' *Pickwick Papers*, the girls, in an interesting androgynous action, took on the male names and characters of those who made up Mr. Pickwick's group of traveling comic figures. Maida's pseudonym was Tracy Tupman, a plump middle-aged dandy. Interestingly, so strongly were those assumed identities that eighty years later May Koshland could not remember Maida, but upon seeing her ejaculated, 'Tracy Tupman!'"
10 Oral Memoir, 1:24
11 Jabberwock, 21, no. 8 (May 1908), Girls' Latin School, Boston, MA.

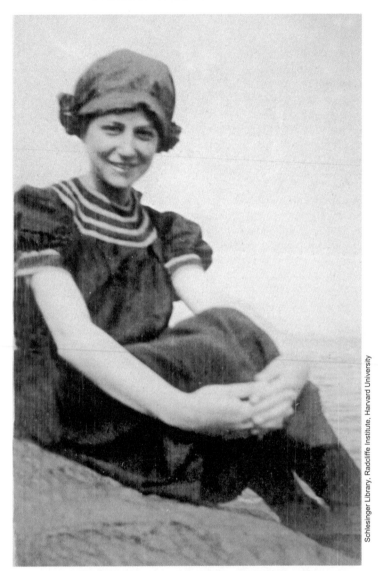

Schlesinger Library, Radcliffe Institute, Harvard University

Maida Herman, age 18, a Smith College student
at the beach, Lynn, MA, summer 1909.

2

The Smith Years

The five members of the Pickwick Club attended either Girls' Latin School or a finishing school called Miss May's. All had plans to go on to college. Fanny Frank, a cousin of Maida's, went on to Radcliffe where she attended for two years, before deciding to enter social work by becoming a volunteer at the Massachusetts General Hospital. "She went and did volunteer work there. By then I was in college and she would write me about the work she was doing as a volunteer."[1]

Helen Strauss, a Pickwick Club member, was planning to go to Smith, as was May Koshland. Maida had no intention of following her sister Bess to Radcliffe and commuting to school as she had done to Girls' Latin School. Bess helped Maida influence their father to allow Maida to break new ground and go off to Smith as well. A teacher at Girls' Latin, Abby C. Howes, was a Smith graduate and apparently thought that her alma mater would be a good choice for Maida.[2] Her friends were a powerful influence on her choice. At Smith May and Maida lived in different houses. Their parents thought "separation was wise…since we should not all be in the same house…too many Jewish girls in one house," they said, but May stayed at Smith only one year.[3]

There may have been another factor in Maida's father's decision to allow his youngest daughter to go away to school: Bess's report of religious discrimination then at Radcliffe. Perhaps the Hermans were trying to protect their daughter from religious intolerance at college. But in seeking to protect her from it, they also helped set in motion a process of development that started her on a journey toward greater independence and maturity.

Her enthusiasm for this new phase of her life is reflected in her detailed notes in her diary of April 25, 1908:

Grandest most gorgeous day! I'm so excited, delighted, happy. Mother, Helen and I went to Smith!! Victor Greenbaum has a girl friend up there, Helen Kramer...he telephoned her we were coming, told her to meet us at the station. He took us to the station...9:15 train. Boston and Albany. Arrived at Springfield at 11:40. Took train—arrived at Northampton at 12:30—nice trip. Helen Kramer met us...she was with us from 12:30 to 5:41. She showed us the store, tearoom, then we went to Helen's room and met her roommate...Their rooms! Heaven, dandy study, bully bedroom. Met two other girls...then we went room hunting. The spirit up there is great, you walk into girls' rooms when you want and they're happy and nice. We went to Mlle. Vincens 75 West...bully house—may give us single rooms, then to Henshaw Place.

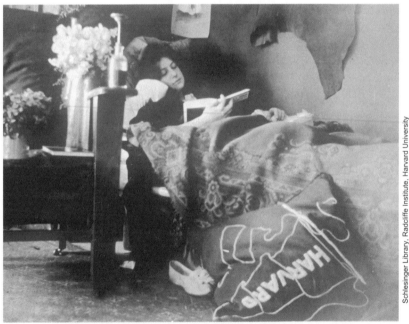

Maida Herman reading in bed at Smith College
on her 19th birthday, March 9, 1910.

Mrs. Hogland intends to open a new house…30 girls, West St.—then to Green St.—can get a double room. Went to other houses…no rooms. Walked around. Had a healthy, happy time…Then we went to the Copper Kettle tearoom. Saw the campus…Came home…arrived at Springfield 6:15, left at 7:14, arrived Boston 9:30.[4]

In a note dated June 3, 1908, Maida wrote, "Helen (Strauss) and I have rooms [at Smith] in the French House…she has #19, I, #17." On September 11 she wrote, "Helen isn't going to college. She's going to study music. My sorrow is untold."[5]

On Tuesday, September 15, 1908, Maida, accompanied by her mother, traveled to Smith to begin her freshman year. Upon arrival, she met other new residents of the French House, "Luella McNay… awfully sweet; Ethel Scarefe…western and full of fun; Adele Peterson…bright, talented and fun." Her diary records her first days at college:

> September 16, unpacked all morn; met Louise Benjamin [who] lives next door with Edna Dunham.
> September 17, went to Chapel…Mother left this morning. I felt awfully but I didn't cry as she went out. Attended President's lecture at 11, then at two o'clock met my advisor and arranged my courses: Latin, German, French, Math, English, and the weekly President's lecture.[6]

Additional requirements were daily attendance at chapel, as well as Bible studies and vespers.

Maida greatly valued her four years at Smith. She always thought of herself as a Smith woman, stating that it was a "frightfully important thing." She wrote in her diary:

> I valued it very much because I loved it…loved the country…some of the teachers…and the idea that I could work at whatever I wanted to. I enjoyed it. When I went to work afterwards, and would announce that I went to Smith, at that time they wouldn't believe that a college woman would want to work, etc., and at one time, I brought in my diploma and I always cared about it. I've kept it around. I know where it is. I've always belonged to the Smith clubs and I've always gone back to reunions even as I become more and more accepted as a Jewish, professional American woman.[7]

Maida had strong ideas about what was important for her to do as a woman and these were nurtured at Smith. What has stood as perhaps Maida's outstanding personal hallmark was her strong sense of independence.

> I was clear that I wanted to marry, that I wanted to have a career, that I wanted to have children, and I wanted to combine them all...[This was in 1912]. I also felt that...believed, rather, that women were equal to men and that I was equal to any man whom I knew...in ability, in power to make my own decisions in regard to work, life and sex![8]

Along with her studies, Maida began an avid, lifelong interest in both individual and competitive team sports. She played in tennis tournaments, rode horses, ice-skated, and canoed. She was a member of the cricket team and basketball team. As a freshman she enjoyed an active social life as well, writing descriptively of parties and dances she attended, commenting on the clothing, food, and surroundings:

> My room is thought the prettiest in the house. It has a red rug, green wallpaper. My lovely Europe pictures hang on the walls...in one corner I have a poster. I have three windows opposite a door. In the left corner, lovely desk with beautiful desk set, etc. on it. Then closet, then thing for food with chafing dish, then door, then book case, then the other wall, couch, shirt-waist box, then in corner a screen behind which is a chair and chiffonnier. In middle is a Morris chair and two other chairs.[9]

In her diary for October 3, 1908, Maida wrote of her freshman year: "I haven't been very homesick, just once in a great while. I feel I am going to benefit from this college life in many ways."

In a letter to her brother-in-law, Jim Rosenberg, Maida wrote glowingly and insightfully of her first semester at Smith:

> The spirit of the college appeals to me most; it is so wholesome, kind, self-denying and generous. So very much good can be derived from it. The atmosphere is friendly. There is a lot of dandy fun which I love as it is so new. The whole ensemble is alluring and refreshing after narrow Boston...I'm so glad I came here and want to stay. After college I'd love to go to Europe to study. One month in Germany for the language, four in Paris for everything and two in Italy. Wouldn't that be divine?

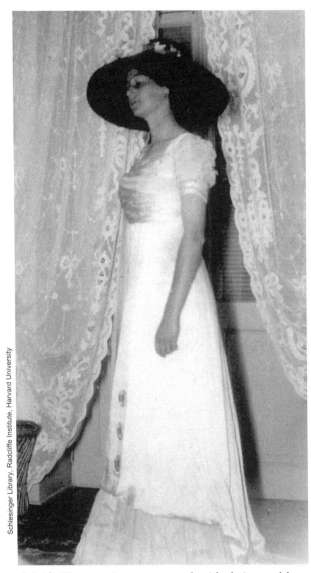

Maida Herman in a gown and wide-brimmed hat
during her junior year at Smith College, 1911.

She also wrote that after her trip to Europe she would like to return to Boston and, at 21, become engaged. Any idea of who her fiancé might be was left unstated; in fact, she had not yet met her future husband.

Of her studies she wrote:

> I do them as decently as I did in the Latin School, but don't spend more than an hour on any [two being required], except on Math and English...the one because I loathe it, the other because I love it. If I spent full time I'd make brilliant translations but I'd rather train myself to quickness, not waste so much time and have more pleasure in life. I am

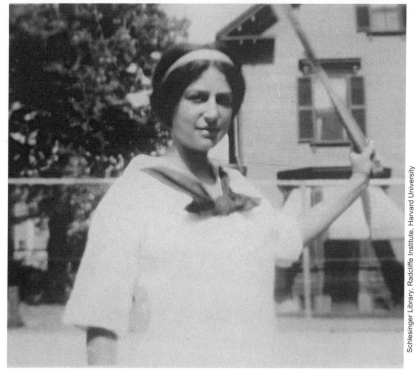

Maida Herman, Charlestown Navy Yard, 1912.
(In 1975, age 84, Maida was still playing tennis.)

systematic and can concentrate and do a thing when I sit down to it, not remaining with a book unopened…I had a beautiful time this after[noon] doing English. I made an outline of the Pathetic Fallacy…which is bully and read Wordsworth and Sheridan in connection with it. Now I like stuff like that, but pesky planes, polygons, polyhedrons, pentagons, prisms, pyramids, may this collection of 'p's' go to H…!

I'm a little disappointed in French but hope it will be more thrilling later on. I am passionately joyful over our weekly art class and expect to learn a heap from it. The Bible class does not fill me with quite as much enthusiasm, but I realize it's worthwhile and fairly interesting. I didn't go last week, stayed home and wrote poems for Helen instead.

I love to finish my work, get it out of the way and when it is finished I promptly put it out of my mind and don't bother about it.

Of her first-term exams she writes, "Sunday, January 31…I passed well in Math, quite well in English, 'A' in Latin, quite well in French."

In her sophomore year Maida described her social life in Boston: the letters, telegrams, flowers, and candy she received from a number of beaux, as well as the men she met through her classmates. She accepted a number of invitations to dances, theater, and dinner, going back between Boston, New York, and Washington, DC.

Maida's oldest sister Sara married Sol Barnet on February 18, 1909. Maida went home to Boston for the wedding. She was very excited about it, delighted to be an important participant. "Sara, Bess and I had our last walk while she was unmarried." She wrote:

Came home and had my hair dressed at 5—$2. It was in puffs and two roses put in gracefully. Supper at 5:30. Put rice in the suitcase. Sara left and Burnsie came and dressed us. My dress was simply beautiful, long pink stuff starting at the bust…the dress was absolutely simple. Nothing on it at all. From one shoulder was sort of a sash, then tulle, with goldish cloth buttons. It was low neck and my bones didn't show. Sara was quiet getting dressed and made a lovely, beautiful bride…the ceremony was nice…it really was a divine wedding…everything lovely…danced all evening, got to sleep about 4:30. I couldn't be too sad as Sara was so happy and Sol is such a peach.[10]

In her early years at Smith, Maida remained close to her old friends from the Pickwick Club. During a spring vacation, Maida noted in her diary on Sunday, March 26, "Evening Pickwick dinner at Fan's." She looked forward to seeing her friend Helen Strauss, a Pickwick member in Paris with her parents, a few days later. But it was her family that continued to figure most in Maida's early college influences. Tuesday, March 9, 1909, was her first birthday celebrated at Smith College:

> My 18th birthday! Went down to breakfast and found red pinks from Moo [Mother]. Got 11 letters...stayed and cut part of Latin [class] to read them...Went to Springfield [MA] to meet Moo, found Foo [Father] there for a surprise. It poured so we went to my room and lots of

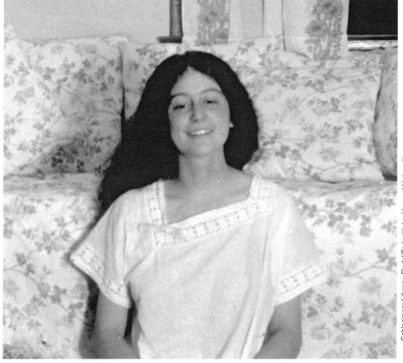

Maida Herman in her dormitory room, 1912.

girls, flowers, presents came. We went back to see Foo, then dinner at Boydens. Telephone from May; cablegram from Helen…I stayed up 'til 12:30 writing and gazing at my presents…Thackeray, pin, diamond ring from Moo, Kipling from Aunt Lina, racquet from Sophie, flowers from Helen, Mildred, Edna, Louise and Irene etc., 6 telegrams, 17 letters.[11]

Maida's pleasure in marking her birthdays continued throughout her life. They became an annual celebration with her social work colleagues as well as her family.

A letter from Maida's father written a day later indicates the depth and tenderness of his feeling for his youngest offspring and his hopes for her future:

> My dear Maida,
>   Enjoyed my day with you very much, firstly because you appear to be so happy in your surroundings, which impresses me in a measure for the large sacrifice it has incurred me in letting you go away from home, but also in having been an eye witness to the happy 18th birthday which you just celebrated. I expect a good many great things from you and I know you will not disappoint me; you know I do not say much, but I think a great lot.
>   Enclosed find a little present which I intended to give you this morning, but was afraid your mother would have kicked, thinking I am spoiling you…maybe she is right, but I take my chances. Nothing else for today, with ever so much love from…
>
> Your loving and devoted Father

But this parental support and closeness became something with which Maida and her family would soon have to contend. Maida's horizons expanded both on and off the campus, particularly in her senior year at Smith. During this period, 1911-1912, Maida became a member of the Massachusetts Women's Suffrage Association (annual dues $1.00). When she moved into Northrop, a new house on campus that became home during her senior year, she met some men outside of college at the People's Institute, where she taught English to Russian immigrants. There she met people who gave their time to teaching and were an influence on Maida's thinking about her future career, as well as about how she might contribute to the community. "They were interested in women being important and me, one of them!"[12] she wrote.

The idea of well-off women wanting to support themselves by having a paid job outside of the home, however, was something that never occurred to Maida's parents. "My parents had no idea I would ever want to do any work. It wasn't expected." It was the expectation that women would marry after graduation, "and some of us intended to work and marry, both!"[13]

When Maida graduated on Sunday, June 18, 1912, the educator and critic Bliss Perry delivered a commencement address on "Fellowship and Individuality." Earlier her mother had written her: "Well, my dearest girl, you have had a fun, happy, carefree as well as instructive and interesting time at your beloved college and I know that you are sad at thoughts of leaving your beloved Alma Mater...You are now to take your place in the world and I know you will come home to be with your old Foo and Moo with a happy heart. I hope these last days [at school] will be full of joy and happiness for my baby girl."

Maida had been steeped in the tradition of social service exemplified by the Hechts (Aunt Lina and Uncle Jake), and transmitted by her parents. It was a tradition in the family, part of the milieu in which she had grown up. But she was also still part of the broader milieu in which her parents proudly had been able to raise her, still subject to their expectations and to those of the wider world with respect to women in general and women of her class and status in particular. It was not easy for her to sort out what to embrace and build on and what to contend with or fight against and change in this multifaceted cultural heritage. What she wanted, as she later put it,

> ...was to make my contribution and do it my way. What I wanted to do [after graduation] was to go on in social work...and the reason I didn't do it right away, was [my] resistance to the family tradition...because of my mother, who was still extremely active in all those organizations and so was my father...and because I just wanted to be separated from them both in my interests and physically. I wanted to leave home, that was quite clear...but I couldn't manage it.

Maida and her roommate went up to Woodstock, New Hampshire and spent a week "facing the problem...of going home," she recalled. In her diary she wrote, "Fri. June 21, first day at N. Woodstock. Wrote 16 notes in the morn—freezing—fire—walked a bit. Slept 2–5. Unpacked trunk, walked in eve—talked of our future—families. Both cried."[14]

A loving and supportive letter from her sister Bess, dated that same day, beginning "Dearest Kidlet," shows the emotional and intellectual conflicts with which Maida struggled at this time. Bess had seen Maida's agitation when the family attended graduation ceremonies at Smith:

> Shall I tell you what I noticed? Well—I noticed that mother somewhat got on your nerves and that, tho she understands a lot, she doesn't live in your aspirations and ideals. Her nature is too different and it probably annoys you to have her fuss over details when you're thinking of 'big' things. Then I noticed as always, the very (to me) pathetic, struggling

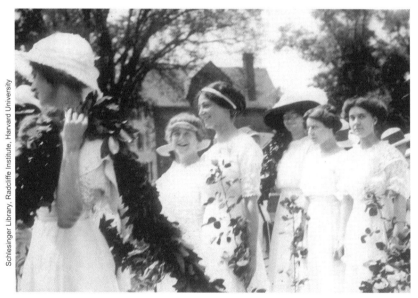

Maida Herman (center, holding long flower stem) during her commencement ceremonies at Smith College, June 1912.

opposition of Father. He...won't understand modern girlhood in the form of his daughter. I sometimes think that he sympathizes and is totally unable to show his feelings. Coming away from Ivy Exercises he said to us, 'When I heard that girl [the orator] talk I saw what college life means to those girls.' Now I don't think he would have said that to you. Do you?...

Father certainly deserves our love and our endeavor to make him happy. You may say you are young and have your own life to lead. But it's just because you're young and have all of life before you that I ask this of you. Father is old and his life has not been happy from your and my point of view. He did not have the advantage of education or leisure to help him understand and enjoy his children. He gives us love and caresses and all we ask for are presents and money, but he can't give you the sympathy you want because his nature and his life have withheld from him the power. He has yielded you the big point of letting you work. Remember that and don't take it for granted, for it was a hard step for him.

You told me that struggle would come in a year and you mean leaving home by that. Now listen. When you wrote that, I felt you were right, that if you wanted to go, you had the right and in a way, you have. But why should you go? You have no special call anywhere else at present. My point is this. Either you don't marry and have all of life before you to do as you like, and in that case, these 5 or 10 years won't matter as you can train for any sort of work in Boston...or, which is more likely, you do marry in time. How much happier will your whole future life be if you've done your duty and made your father's and others' lives content instead of embittered...

Remember your baccalaureate sermon. We cannot live for ourselves alone. So far, you've had all you've asked for and have gotten those wonderful years at college, through Father and without any opposition. Now remember that you are part of a family and that doing right by them is a good beginning for doing your share toward society and the world.

Maida's sister speaks her advice in the voice of her time and place, a voice that can be heard speaking in louder tones in a letter from her brother-in-law, Jim:

Bess read me your letter [possibly in reply to the above] and an extraordinarily well-reasoned, logical, clear and in many respects, a soundly analyzed document it seems to me. Now I am not, except by the kind adoption of Bess, a member of your family. So that I have the advantage of being the intelligent observer who can get off far enough to have a perspective and can see the thing in its more general relation to life at large...

In conceding to you the vital importance of your next 5 to 10 years, your right to your own life, your development of your own individuality, your formation of your own lines of thinking and doing, I feel that your duty is to stay at home and that to do so is in the truest sense the way to see your own visions, live your own life, wage your own battles...

Do you seek to go into social service work, to take a secretarial position, to go into business in one form or another? Where would you look, but in a big city? Staying at home can be made by you to mean what staying at home means to any business or professional man. It is his place of rest, peace, refuge. There are those we love and while that love is an ampler thing than the love of the child for the parent, yet the principles are the same...

Life is just seething 'round you in Boston. Jobs on newspapers, in bookstores, teaching jobs, charity work, social service work—everything is there that you can find anywhere. And believe me when you come home tired after a day's work, 424 Marlboro and a father and mother sympathetic and interested—they will be, I'm sure of it—will be better than an $8.00 a week boarding house. For if you do strike out away from everyone you won't let your father pay the bills, I suppose—and if you get a job at more than $20.00 a week you'll be wonderful. So chew it over, and don't fret.

Your loving (adopted) brother, Jim

With such advice ringing in her ears, Maida faced the "problem of going home."

Notes to Chapter 2: The Smith Years

1 Quoted from: Maida Herman Solomon Oral Memoirs, American Jewish
Committee, 3 volumes, Oral Memoir, 1:18-19.
2 ibid., 1:38
3 ibid., 1:22
4 Diary, Maida Herman, April 25, 1908
5 ibid., September 11, 1908
6 Oral Memoir, 1:56
7 ibid., 1:66
8 ibid., 1:69-70
9 Diary, October 3, 1908
10 ibid., 113-119
11 ibid., 130-132
12 Oral Memoir, 1:59-63
13 ibid., 61, 59
14 ibid., 1:72-73, 68-69

3
Transitions

The years from 1914 to 1916 were "transitional," as Maida recalled them. "They were the years in which I worked in my first permanent paid employment prior to marriage," she wrote, "and expressed openly an affiliation with Jewish organizations…some important to the family and other newer groups in which I participated as a young college graduate."[1]

Those transitional years included her marriage, on June 27, 1916, to Dr. Harry Caesar Solomon. During this period Maida was able to work through many of the questions and conflicts that had been troublesome to her.

In her diary Maida stated, "[We'd] talked of our future and that I would work and that we'd have babies and that I'd be a wife. I'd combine the three of them and he agreed."[2] This brief but profound statement was to become a hallmark of her life's journey!

Although she had hoped for an alternative to a return to Boston and her family, Maida began considering her options prior to her graduation, but those options did not seem encouraging. In the spring of her senior year she had asked for information about the secretarial program at Simmons Female College, now Simmons College. The director of the appointment bureau of the Women's Educational and Industrial Bureau in Boston had written:

> Thank you for your registration which we have received this morning. Although the year's course at Simmons undoubtedly gives the best training, it is possible to get stenographic positions after two or three months' training at a business school. We have calls sometimes that ask definitely for a college girl with Simmons training. You, of course,

would not be eligible for such a position if you had not been at Simmons.

Maida also inquired at the Hickox Shorthand School of Boston and received the following information from Mr. William Hickox, describing the future that a young woman with a Smith education could aspire:

> The shorter course (session nine to twelve o'clock) tuition [is] twelve dollars a month, [and] is designed for those who do not find it practicable to give their entire time to study. The full course, at fifteen dollars a month, is from nine to two…The subjects exclusively taught are Touch Typing, of which this school is a pioneer, Pitman's Phonography, modernized and simplified by the principal, and English, with special reference to preparing for high-grade secretarial positions. Competent pupils, past and present, whether graduates or not, are placed in lucrative employment by the school when desired.

Maida was seriously planning for her future as a working woman. After careful research into various programs, with the blessing of her family and to their great relief, Maida chose to matriculate at Simmons Female College the following September and enrolled in their secretarial program on September 22, 1912. There she learned stenography and typing. "By the time we got through we were prepared to be secretaries, not stenographers, but secretaries with all those extra skills." And according to Simmons at that time… "We had to do six months' practical work."[3]

It was at that time still her intention to work at something other than the family calling—she was determined to work in the field of social service, and she intended to get the necessary training for it. She studied "business, law, and accounting," which she found quite useful.

But if she was preparing for the inevitable fate of a young woman of her education and class in the workplace of the day, she was not submitting to it. Maida's life during the next two years was extremely busy with activities that took her well beyond her vocational plans: she took drama at Boston University and continued her interest in tennis, swimming, skating, travel, and volunteer work. She enrolled at the Portia School of Law in the evening.

I couldn't get in anywhere else because I was a woman…I went around [to various schools]…I went to the Harvard Law School, and I was going, at that time, with somebody who was a graduate of the Harvard Law School…and I was influenced by that, and he found out that I couldn't go. I used all his law books and found them very useful, and I took contracts and torts…I went two evenings a week and I found that knowledge useful to me.[4]

During these years one of the ways in which Maida began to work out her concerns was by developing her own ways of carrying on the family's tradition of social service and social action. Like the Hechts and her parents, she found the synagogue an institution ready and willing to lend intellectual support to these ongoing concerns.

One of Maida's consuming interests at this time was the Union Park Forum, an organization formed during the period 1914-1915 (it lasted well into the 1920s) at a meeting at Temple Ohabei Shalom, which was then located in Boston's South End. Frances Stern, "an important figure in my life,"[5] Maida recalled, was one of the people crucial to the Forum's inception, and she drew into it Herbert Ehrmann, together with his wife Sarah (who were to become the closest of friends to Maida and Harry), and also Adolph Giesberg, Walter Lippman, John Reed, and the young Maida Herman, to name a few.

Modeled after the Ford Hall Forum, the Union Park Forum provided a place for Jewish people to be able to hear lectures by the prominent intelligentsia of the day. It was open to everyone, which was important to Maida. She explained:

There were a lot of Jewish people who couldn't get into Ford Hall, get there on time, and Frances felt that there was a need in the South End community…it was a great community effort…open to immigrants, residents of the community… and I was very active, extremely active in getting the lecturers…some of whom were Jewish and some of whom were not.[6]

Speakers included the U.S. Supreme Court Justice Felix Frankfurter and Rabbi Stephen Wise (a lifelong friend who later performed the marriage ceremony for Maida and Harry, as well as a few decades later the ceremony of their son Peter and Barbara Miller). Maida also noted that, "Ben Scharff (another long-time friend) took me to Frances Stern's home where there I met Felix Frankfurter and...I got to know Felix Frankfurter quite a bit."[7]

She also knew Louis Kirstein, a family friend who invited Maida to serve on the board of the Jewish Federation, an organization in which Maida's father was one of the prime movers. She was the only young person to serve on the board at that time. As Maida realized, just as her other activities served as a link to her mother and the Hechts, the Federation served as a link with her father.[8] Maida eventually became an active, fifty-year member of the Hecht House Board of Directors, which secured that link to her family's community interests.

In 1915, the suffrage movement also became a main focus of Maida's life. She had been a member since Smith, but now became increasingly active. In November, Maida carried a banner at the head of a suffragists' parade down Tremont Street in Boston. She also became a member of the Council of Jewish Women, an organization with which she kept a lifelong affiliation. In short, during these years Maida became extremely involved in a number of important voluntary community activities in which she held important positions.

Her resistance to putting her own stamp on the traditions of her family and the community were melting away. The work she found assisted in that process; she decided that social work was indeed her destiny. But her first job reminded her that she had not escaped all the problems she faced as she contemplated the possibilities opened to her upon graduating from Smith.

Upon her graduation from Simmons Female College with a Bachelor of Science degree in June 1914, Maida landed her first permanent paid employment at the Civic Service House. Her assignment was to "assist secretarially to Mr. Philip Davis on the research work he was doing on the adolescent boy."

> I took notes and I edited them and wrote things and did a lot of reading and I became sort of a research person...We had some material ready for publication and I guess we had a publisher, I think it was Little

Brown…At any rate, Mr. Davis put my name on the title page 'In collaboration with…' and the head of the project said, 'Your name cannot be there. It can be in a footnote that you've collaborated and everything, but you cannot be down as one of the co-editors or co-authors or co-anything because we don't want another Jewish name (Davis was Jewish), and we don't want a woman.' I left his office that day and I got into the streetcar and I think I drove back and forth forever trying to get rid of my emotions![9]

This episode was intolerable to her: it violated every principle she had. And the book published did in fact recognize Maida Herman as Davis's collaborator.[10] The lesson Maida learned very early in her career was clearly imparted to those of us working under her tutelage some fifty-five years later. Betty Ann Lifson, MSW, recalled that:

She [Maida Solomon] would insist that female psychiatric social workers put their names and titles (and dates) on everything they wrote. Up until this time, female social workers were apt to have written chapters for books and articles or parts of articles to which they would not sign their name or date or stamp 'Not for Publication' and would stand by passively to see their work published under the byline of some male physician or psychologist or sociologist, with maybe a footnote thanking them for their 'help.'

Prior to the publication of *The Field of Social Service* in 1915, Maida spent two years investigating the problem of the adolescent boy in the home, school, industry, etc., at the Civic Service House. Under the auspices of the National Foundation of Settlements, the job required attending various interesting conferences in different cities. At the American Social Hygiene Conference in 1915, Maida's boss, Philip Davis, received a $3,000 contract from Julia Lathrop, then director of the Children's Bureau. The contract enabled him to hire Maida as a full-fledged research assistant. Out of this research came an article by Maida: "The Boy Problem," published in the proceedings of the National Conference on the Education of the Dependent Delinquent and Backward Children, 1915.[11]

At the same time, Maida's professional and intellectual life was beginning to coalesce around the field of social work. Her own social life, from the Union Park Forum to "tea dancing at the Copley Plaza," was bringing her into contact with several eligible bachelors among the Boston/Cambridge Jewish intelligentsia. She wrote: "Went out with Carl Dreyfus. Lee Simonson and I were violently good friends; Abe Pinanski (a Russian Jewish friend who eventually became a Superior Court Judge) and I went out a good deal to the Harvard Club in

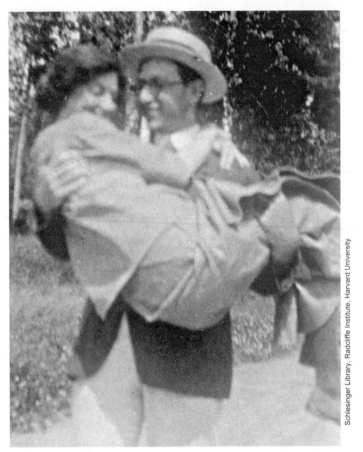

Maida Herman Solomon, bride, in the arms of her husband, Dr. Harry Solomon, Rangeley Lake, Maine, summer 1916.

1914...he tutored me in the law...he brought over his books from Harvard...he was a serious person, he like me seriously."[12] Others she saw socially during this period included Horace Kallen, a Ph.D. in philosophy, later a famous educational theorist on the faculty at the New School for Social Research, and Edwin Cohen, later a professor in biology at the Harvard Medical School.

She also noted in her diary of March 1914, "A Mr. Solomon [at the time at Harvard Medical School] walked me home." She added, "March 27, 1914: Harry Solomon to supper, good time."[13]

A number of her Smith friends were becoming engaged and married, and Maida attended their weddings in Boston, New York, and Baltimore. Although she was seeing others as well, she began to attend symphony concerts with Harry. In September they went to the Touraine Hotel for dinner and the theater, and to a "rather fun" dinner-dance at Temple Israel. In the last entry of her diary, on April 19, 1915, Maida wrote, "I gave H [Harry] an answer. We gradually got to the point of talking to Moo and Foo and announced our engagement April 27, 1915. Picture in the paper. I was excited. Apartment hunting. Adore it. No ring. Don't want one."

Fourteen months later a Boston newspaper announced:

 Miss Maida Herman, daughter of Mr. and Mrs. Joseph M. Herman, of 424 Marlborough St., became the wife of Dr. Harry C. Solomon of Los Angeles, California, at a brilliant wedding at the Somerset [Hotel] last evening. A dinner with three hundred guests followed.

With Harry, Maida had made her first visit to the Boston Psychopathic Hospital, "the Psycho"* as it was affectionately called, and with him she attended the first of many staff meetings there. "I guess that was my first feeling for psychiatric social work, in 1915," she would say.[14]

In April 1916, two months before her marriage, Harry again took Maida to the Boston Psychopathic Hospital, this time to meet Mary Jarrett, who served as its social work department's first director. "It's at that time that I was moving...Harry was moving me, my husband-to-be, toward working over to that aspect of social work, that is, psychiatric social work."[15] **

Harry Solomon at the time was working for the state as head of therapeutic research dealing with neurosyphilitic patients. "Mary Jarrett talked to my husband," Maida recounts, "and felt it was important that these particular patients should have a social worker working with them, who were mostly men, with their wives and with their children."

> She [Miss Jarrett] had nobody to provide for that. She raised some money and she thought I would be a good person to take that on. I became interested in mental hygiene [in a psychiatric setting], in patients,

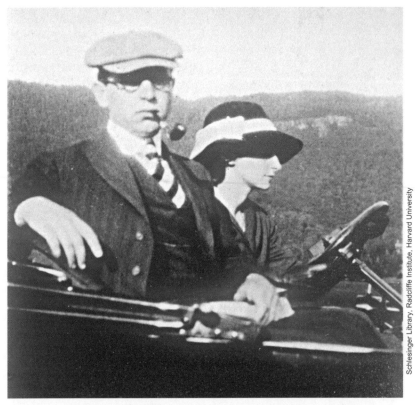

Maida Solomon chauffering her husband, Dr. Harry Solomon,
Dixville Notch, New Hampshire, 1916.

in people, as I had gone over quite a few times with my husband to the hospital and had seen patients and the kind of work the social workers were doing, so I thought it was a very good opportunity to move my interests into the field of mental hygiene, as it was called then, and social work.

The term 'psychiatric social work' was invented, one might say, by Dr. Southard, the head of the hospital, and by Miss Jarrett, at the time I was there during those two years [1916-1918]...Miss Jarrett took me on as an untrained person. It was the pattern in the Boston vicinity and other places for people...young educated women to give of their time and efforts for pay or very often as volunteers...and to receive what is now known, and really perhaps was known, as 'on-the-job-training.'

Miss Jarrett herself had not graduated from a school of social work and neither had her two main associates at that time. The focus of my work became an open-ended one. My husband was interested in research. I had been doing research. I saw there was an opportunity to continue that.[16]

Miss Jarrett established a training program for her workers. Maida became one of eight women who received daily in-service training on what part the social worker would play in the lives of patients and their families, as well as what their responsibilities as staff members in the context of a psychiatric setting would be. Maida determined that she was "a bit more interested in research, and in the education angle [as differentiated from direct clinical service]."[17]

Training and research were to remain her special areas of professional excellence and expertise throughout her life.

It was very easy for me to fall into the picture of research and training...I could see mental illness very clearly, both on an in-patient and out-patient basis. I saw syphilis at that time as one of the main causes of mental illness in untreated men and that became one of my main interests.[18]

Maida elaborated:

My special interest was the families of these people who had a specific illness...the specific illness involved a great deal because syphilis was a social 'disease' and you didn't talk about it, you didn't write about it, et-cetera, and I became interested then in sharing with the general public the fact that syphilis was something that could be acquired and one shouldn't be ashamed of, and in all of this I was very influenced by my husband, who was the head of this little team, consisting of husband and wife.[19]

Maida later recalled,

Studies were a part of Mary Jarrett's vision for psychiatric social work and certainly when I went to the hospital at this time to work under my husband, his interest was [both the] treatment of patients and families, then research, and so my training came from both sides; social work and psychiatry.[20]

Miss Jarrett was able to raise some money from the Carter Ink Company for Maida's modest full-time salary of $75 per month/$900 a year. "I worked full-time and I went to work at eight-thirty and came back whenever I got through, at five-thirty. I had no children and it was just a question of my husband's and my relationship, and it was during this period that I was often left alone because he worked in the evening."

Dr. Shore described Maida's work thusly:

At the Psychiatric Hospital she was a research social worker in the division of Research on Brain Syphilis, headed by her husband, Harry C. Solomon. She followed up patients with the disease, interviewed their contacts and their families, and took a special interest in their children who developed congenital syphilis.

Stunned as we are by the current epidemic of AIDS, we struggle to remember the deadly precedent set by syphilis. It was widespread in the population at that time and was a major cause of mental illness. Although present in Western Europe since the fifteenth century, its cunning and varied guises had not been collected as due to one illness until the nineteenth century and the offending organism was not identified until 1905.

Salvarsan, Paul Ehrlich's famous 'magic bullet,' which for the first time provided reliable, specific treatment, was developed only in 1909 or 1910.

The title of Maida and Harry Solomon's report on their collaborative work, *Syphilis of the Innocent*, reminds us of that terrible time and the effect of syphilis on families and urban children.[21]

Maida became a pioneer in the education of psychiatric social workers as a result of her work at the Boston Psychopathic Hospital. By the fall of 1918, Mary Jarrett, Frank Wood Williams, Dr. Elmer Southard, and the heads of Smith College "conceived the idea of training psychiatric social workers. All of us there worked with Miss Jarrett on any possible adaptation of the course she was already giving us."[22] It was this course, Maida later stated, that "allowed me to go ahead as a psychiatric social worker."[23]

The Smith College Training School of Psychiatric Social Work began as an emergency program designed to equip social workers with special skills to meet the emergency psychiatric needs of patients in army and civilian hospitals. In 1919, it became the Smith College School for Social Work. The staff and students at the Boston Psychopathic Hospital also had the benefit of the material being presented to all the Harvard medical students by Drs. Southard, Adler, Solomon, Thom, and Myerson.

Between 1916 and 1918, several social work students, probably from Simmons, already had come to "the Psycho" for their training, and later, after the establishment of the Smith school, students from Smith spent a year there as well.

Maida thus learned very early in her career the importance of integrating the theory of the classroom with the practice of the clinical setting. She would foster this hallmark of social work education all her life.

Maida remained at her job for about a year and a half, from September 1916 to March 1918. Harry told her soon after they were married that he was going into the army as a volunteer; that he planned to enlist rather than be drafted. He was called in March 1918 and was assigned to Cape May, New Jersey. At Cape May, Maida learned that she would not be allowed to follow her husband to the European theater. Maida and Harry made their decision together. As she explained, "These things were always joint decisions…that if I wasn't going with him, I was going to have a baby, and so God was with me and I became pregnant."[24]

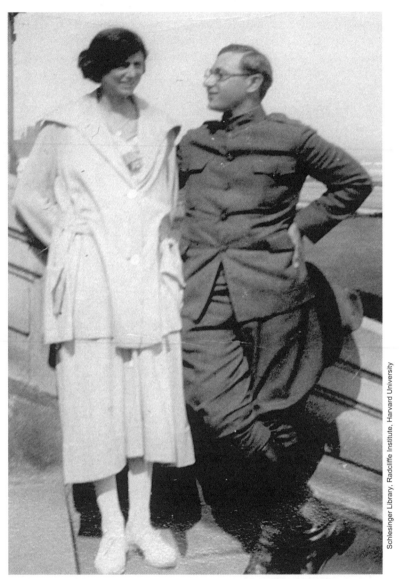

Schlesinger Library, Radcliffe Institute, Harvard University

Maida Solomon with her husband, Dr. Harry Solomon,
U.S. Army, Cape May, New Jersey, March 1918.

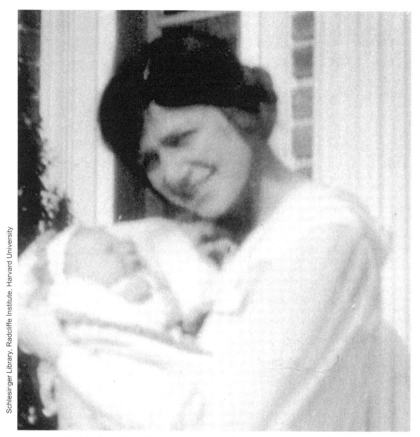

Maida holding her first child, Peter Herman Solomon,
born September 6, 1918.

Harry left for France and Maida returned to Boston to her parents'
home, where their first son, Peter, was born.[25] Because of the epidemic
of often-fatal influenza, Maida stayed in her apartment with the baby,
venturing out only once a week with Peter in tow to lunch with her
mother. An old family retainer who had been in Aunt Lina's service
came to take care of the baby, living with Maida throughout Harry's ab-

sence. "The whole husband/wife team working-child relationship had a strong tie to the fact that in those days we had domestic service."[26]

In the fall of 1918, after Harry's return from France, Maida returned to part-time work at "the Psycho." She was paid for her collaboration as a writer of *Syphilis of the Innocent,* and for acting as a research consultant.

Later, she would work at times as a volunteer. In doing so, she felt strongly that her professionalism was not denigrated. In fact, she felt that she had greater flexibility in shaping her career and its endeavors as a professional volunteer or volunteer professional than she would have had on a set career track.

She was later instrumental in developing professionals who had goals similar to hers and in eventually creating part-time employment opportunities for a large number of professionally trained social workers. So too, she would later develop significant roles for volunteers.

Notes to Chapter 3: Transitions

1 Oral Memoir, 1:88
2 Diary, p. 164
3 Oral Memoir, 1:75
4 ibid., 1:85-86
5 ibid., 1:86
6 ibid., 1:145-148
7 ibid., 1:136-137
8 ibid., 1:139
9 ibid., 1:92-94
10 ibid., 1:106-108
11 Smith College Decennial Yearbook: Class of 1912, 45.
12 Oral Memoir, 1:144
13 Diary, P. 120-124
14 Oral Memoir, 1:142
15 ibid., 1:160
16 Oral Memoir, 1: 160-168
17 ibid., 1:169
18 ibid., 1:174
19 ibid., 1:169-170
20 ibid., 2:238

21 Shore, Miles F., from a speech at a memorial for Maida H. Solomon, MMHC, March 30, 1988.
22 ibid., 1:173-174
23 ibid., 2:238
24 ibid., 1:76
25 see Family Tree, prepared by David Solomon
26 ibid., 1:182

*The Boston Psychopathic Hospital was renamed The Massachusetts Mental Health Center in 1956 during Harry Solomon's "watch" as superintendent. He was also the Bullard Professor of Psychiatry at the Harvard Medical School. Later he was appointed Commissioner of Mental Health of the Commonwealth of Massachusetts.
**For a fascinating account of the early days at the Boston Psychopathic Hospital, see Lunbeck, Elizabeth, "The Psychiatric Persuasion, Knowledge, Gender and Power in Modern America," chapter six—Institutional Discipline, pages 152-181 and pictures immediately following the chapter.

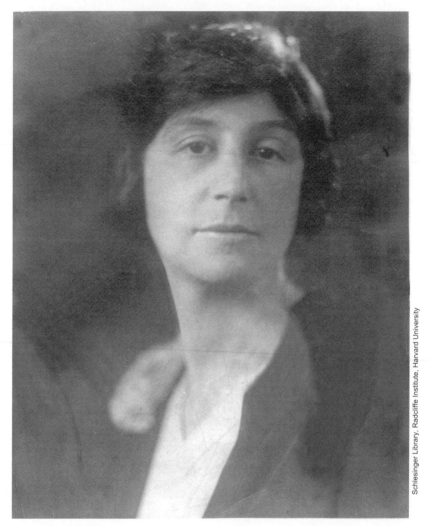

A serious young married woman, Maida Herman Solomon, c. 1916.

4
Psychiatric Social Work

As a psychiatric social worker at the Boston Psychopathic Hospital, Maida learned that a key step in problem-solving included the recording of a detailed social, physical, personal, family and legal history from parents, families, and agencies, as described by Southard and Jarrett in the book, *The Five Kingdoms of Evils*.[1] That book classified social problems as poverty, disease, ignorance, legal issues, and juvenile delinquency. To bring all of these under the umbrella of life difficulties to be treated together from a psychological perspective was revolutionary; Maida and Harry were the first generation of young trainees who did so.

Freud's theory was sweeping the country and had a dramatic impact on social work education and practice:

> [Freud's] perspective refocused the social worker's lens from poverty to the person who was poor, and from social problems like desertion and alcoholism to the individual personalities who were beset by them…Psychoanalytic theory helped transform a one-dimensional moralistic approach to human beings in trouble into a non-judgmental psychosocial process…[Furthermore Freudian psychology] demonstrated how the client's past experiences contributed in a major way to current malfunctioning…psychoanalytic theory enabled social workers to realize that not only were external pressures major contributing factors in their clients' psychosocial problems, but also were internal pressures, such as prohibitive superegos, weak ego functioning, and unresolved infantile wishes.[2]

The *Encyclopedia of Social Work* sheds an interesting light on the history of this period:

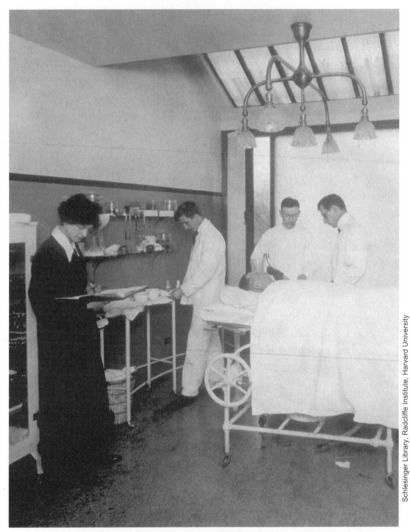

Maida Herman Solomon with appoinment book, and
Dr. Harry Solomon in glasses, treating a syphilitic patient, 1916.

Within a few years, psychiatric caseworkers were firmly established…
the focus on mental health among soldiers in World War I and the dis-
covery of high rates of mental illness among draftees accelerated the
already mushrooming mental health movement, and psychiatric casework, part of the movement almost from the beginning, grew in pace
with it…Since Jarrett and others had already persuaded other caseworkers and some casework educators that psychiatric knowledge was appli-
cable to all casework and should be included in the training of all
caseworkers, Freudian psychology naturally was added in when it began
to permeate the psychiatric field. Thus, increasing numbers of caseworkers could call themselves, if not psychiatric caseworkers, at least
psychiatrically or psychoanalytically 'oriented' in their practice.[3]

Maida was part of, and benefited from, several larger trends—not
only the casework movement, with its distinctly psychiatric side, but
also the so-called "social hygiene" movement that arose in response to
the epidemic of venereal disease. The Massachusetts Social Hygiene
Movement, begun in 1913 by Charles W. Eliot, then president of Harvard, was given impetus in 1915 by Dr. George Bigelow, then superintendent of the Massachusetts General Hospital and later Commissioner
for the Commonwealth of Massachusetts. Once the Solomons' book,
Syphilis of the Innocent, was published under the auspices of the U.S. Department of Social Hygiene, Maida recalled, "I personally began to
know people in the social hygiene movement; so when we had to look
for a statistic, I might get in touch with someone in New York…we
gradually had an interest in this kind of thing."[4]

It was thus that Maida's career interests began to shift in the 1920s
from in-patient psychiatric social work and research to community ac-
tivism and education. When her interest changed, she transferred the
principles she had acquired in one area to fit the needs of her next activity, a pattern she continued throughout her long and illustrious career.
In the Massachusetts Social Hygiene movement she became "a big
boss." She wrote:

It was one of the volunteer things that I picked up from my professional
experience at the Psycho [working on the syphilis study]. I believed that
the knowledge that you have as a professional should be used in the

community...I know I was pregnant at the time [with either Babette, born October, 1924, or Eric, born October, 1928]...I organized and presided at the meetings at the request of Dr. Bigelow, and we tried to put over the idea that we had to educate our young people in the schools to know the meaning of sex, etcetera, etcetera, and that was our effort. It was a successful meeting and it opened areas, and as time went on we were able to secure assistants to Dr. McGillicuddy (a physician and sex educator) and then we moved toward teachers and people interested in schools...Gradually we were able to initiate a meeting with parents...We had some very interesting women working for us...Dr. McGillicuddy was paid (as were others)...All were paid except the officers. I was the vice president. Money was raised through membership dues, and sometimes we got money from American Social Hygiene... Money raising was not anything I enjoyed doing, but once in a while I had to do it.

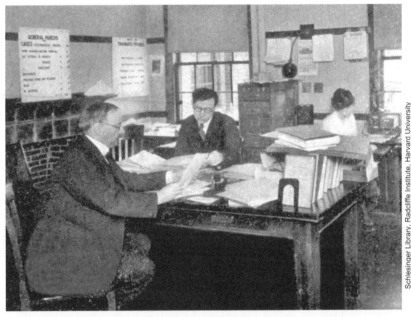

Dr. E. E. Southard, Dr. Harry Solomon, and Maida Solomon, working together on the syphilis project, 1917.

We worked very hard with the Public Health Department because we wanted to have them enforce the law...that you had to have a Wasserman test [prior to marriage]. I remember going to the Public Health Department and offering to get a trained nurse who would go and follow up on the physicians' reports to see whether people really got a Wasserman...That was sort of a research thing to show them that they had to put more people on their staff to get results...They were carrying out my personal research interest there.[5]

Maida served as vice president of the Massachusetts Society for Social Hygiene for twenty-eight years, from 1928 to 1956. During that early period two clinics were started with financial support coming from the Social Hygiene group, in the North End and later in Lowell. Eventually local Boards of Health carried out the work. Maida attended executive meetings where she tried to develop many general policies linking the state society's agenda to that of the American Social Hygiene Association. They published a pamphlet based on her work called *Growing up in the World Today*, which had four printings by 1937.

During this twenty-eight-year period, Maida recalled, "We moved clearly from a public health approach to the educational one...we moved into the schools and really were conscious of the fact that we wanted to give the pupils and the parents and the teachers attitudes; proper attitudes towards sex, knowledge of symptoms of pregnancy, a long way from thinking that VD was a just punishment for sin."[6] The members of the executive committee were very liberal "and would realize clearly that when it was possible one would offer birth control methods...as far as the society was concerned [we] probably wouldn't publicize that too much...[we] would do it quietly and individually...several of us were interested in the Planned Parenthood Association."[7] Elizabeth Lunbeck described a situation thusly:

Maida Solomon related the story of her encounter with an editor of a leading newspaper who, claiming he was catering to a wide and easily offended public, refused to use the word 'syphilis' in his paper's columns. Solomon proposed that the public was enlightened enough 'to at least read the word.' She and other social workers and psychiatrists who dealt with syphilitic patients sketched an ethics of disclosure that was meant to induce patients to speak while at the same time protecting their privacy. This approach promised patients that, in return for speaking frankly, their cases would be handled on a scientific, not a moral, basis. Maintaining that syphilis was neither a moral disease nor a stigma, Solomon stressed that social workers did not 'probe into the method of contraction.'[8]

Maida had a colleague in the Social Hygiene Society who would become increasingly important to her, Eva Whiting White. It was she who was responsible for helping Katherine Hardwick persuade Maida to leave her part-time consultant work at the Psycho and begin teaching at the Simmons College School of Social Work in 1934. Mrs. White was a director and professor at the school and a "favorite" of Maida's. She was one of Simmons' earliest graduates and the head of the Elizabeth Peabody House until she came to the school on a full-time basis, where she taught community organization and group work. Said Maida, "She was very intelligent and was full of initiative. She had great political acumen...and when I got to Simmons...I was exposed again to Mrs. White and her knowledge of the neighborhood." [9]

During the period 1918-1928, Maida gave birth to four children: Peter, Joseph, Babette, and Eric. The children and the entertaining that fell to her husband and her from their two active and professionally distinguished careers made the household a lively one.

Eric, the Solomon's youngest son, recalls his childhood thusly:

> Actually, her life work was very much a part of ours. Every night at dinner (served and provided by the three live-in help—one other, a gardener came by the day), Maida discussed her work adventures, challenges and problems with my father, a superb administrator who provided both solid support and wise counsel. (Reticent to an extreme before his children, he never discussed his work.) Indeed, Maida served as the main communication link between him and us. Interestingly, I never recall them arguing before us, but as my bedroom was next to theirs, I often heard them discussing us late into the night. (He called all the shots.)
>
> By 1938, and for nearly eight years, I was my mother's confidant about Simmons. As a young child, I was brought into her bedroom to play

during her traditional (never broken) 9:00 a.m. breakfast (from a tray in bed), 10:00 bath, dressing, then 10:45 departure for Simmons.

By phone, she spoke to her mother, to Sarah Ehrmann, to her social-work colleague and dear friend Ethel Cohen, and, often, to Frances Stern.

When I was ten, until I graduated from high school, we took a twenty-minute walk most week nights, down the Jamicaway, and she unloaded office politics—Miss Hardwick this, later Mr. Rutherford that, Miss Lloyd…Often she took me to her office and I knew her secretaries (especially Miss Sullivan) well. Many discussions of theses took

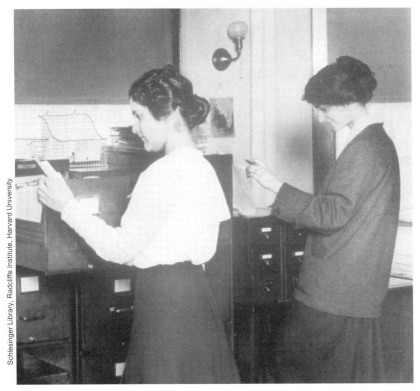

Maida Solomon, right, works with a student volunteer,
Social Work Department, Boston Psychopathic Hospital, 1918.

place, particularly as I became an English teacher. And in her later years, as I became an academic administrator, we discussed how she could, with sensitivity, work as an elder adviser at [the] halfway house and Boston State. And on my quarterly visit in the spring, we discussed prize essays. I was totally drawn into her work life.

Eric also provided a note on the household during these years:

No, she never did an iota of cleaning, cooking (on Sunday nights and after my father cooked), washing, but she did organize servants, hire (most from Antigonish, Nova Scotia) and replace them. She conferred with the cook, from bed, every morning, filling a yearbook with meal plans. (Two servants accompanied us to Maine each summer.)

As a young child, I was cared for by my own nanny. By then, both parents were on the make, and my mother fitted my life and needs into the cracks. That I grew up independent, felt wanted, and never resented (well hardly) absent parents, was testimony to her organizing and affections skills.

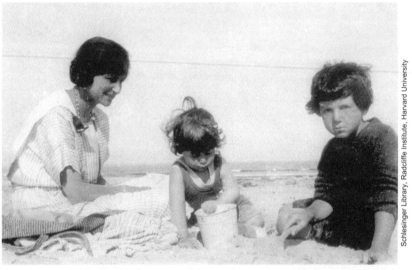

Maida Solomon with her first two children, Joseph (born 1921) and Peter (born 1918), at the beach, 1923.

In 1920 Maida's father died. Mrs. Herman eventually moved from Marlborough Street to the Copley Plaza Hotel, later to the Somerset and then to the Lafayette Hotel. She remained a vital part of activities at the Solomon family home on Lochstead Avenue in Jamaica Plain until her death in 1950.

Eric recalled his grandmother:

> …Visiting for dinner every Tuesday and having most of the family for a hotel Sunday dinner. And Maida spoke by phone to her mother every morning at 9:30. Much of Maida's work ethic emanated from a need to gain approval from this powerful, witty, autocratic, wealthy woman whose other two daughters were respectively, an invalid who died in her forties and a wealthy lawyer's wife.

Meanwhile, Maida was increasingly recognized as a pioneer in the developing field of psychiatric social work. She was a charter member of the American Association of Psychiatric Social Workers (AAPSW) and its first president, 1926-1928. She was a member of its Sub-Committee on Educational Standards and eventually used her work at Simmons to develop national standards for psychiatric social work curricula. She was part of the Temporary Inter-Association Council (TIAC) which planned a single, unified social work organization from specialized groups such as the AAPSW. She was active in the National Association of Social Workers when it was formed in 1955, urging her students to become members.[10]

In the late twenties Maida and Harry were also very involved with the Beth Israel Hospital. They were close friends with many of its leaders and were instrumental in choosing that leadership, thereby helping to lay its foundations of excellence. In 1928 the hospital moved from Townsend Street in Roxbury to its present location on Brookline Avenue, Boston, where it was to become a world-renowned Harvard teaching hospital, a few blocks away from the Harvard Medical School.

The Solomons enjoyed a close friendship with Drs. Harry Linenthal (the four children's pediatrician), Herman Blumgart, and Charles Wilinsky, who were all top men in their respective fields of medicine and who served as members of the executive committee of the Beth Israel Hospital. Dr. Wilinsky later became its director. "We had to get the best people...Jewish or not...Drs. Whittemore and Mixter were not Jewish...but it made no difference."[11]

Maida's interest was in making certain that social work, which had been a part of the Townsend Street facility, would continue to prosper at its new location. Dr. Linenthal called together a committee made up of Maida, Mrs. Nathan Gordon, Mrs. David Small, and Frances Stern. Maida authored a "plan that clearly said that the head social worker should have a master's degree, or the equivalent experience (I think there were two workers we asked for then). It was spelled out in this simple way for the trustees, and then it gave the salary, which to me seems a little mild, but I thought it was quite large at the time and I think it was three thousand [dollars] minimum [for the head social worker]."[12]

The board of trustees was "a group of men [who] had probably never heard of social work really and the idea of professional and master's and everything else... and they passed it and they said that's what it should be. And then it went back to the medical executive commit- tee...Linenthal and everybody, and it was at that time the suggestion was made that Miss Ethel Cohen would be a good person."[13] Maida of- fered the position to Miss Cohen in the spring of 1928, during her sec- ond year at Simmons.

Maida assumed the chair of the Social Service Committee of the Beth Israel Hospital and remained in the position for ten years. The committee established that the director of social service was responsible to Dr. Wilinsky, then head of the hospital. "And that to me was an in- teresting decision because it gave the Social Service Committee and the director of Social Work [Miss Cohen] direct access to Dr. Wilinsky...Our job was the initiating, the changing and the carrying out of social services policies. Now, that's a big order, but that was my concept of my duty as the chairman of the committee."[14]

Maida also viewed the Social Service Committee as a place where the social service director could be backed on issues she saw as needing backing.

And the thing that I was interested in at the time was pushing standards of training and experience of personnel. It was indicated to me by my experience as a worker and working with the Smith School, you had to have training and experience…and it went on to the pushing of active teaching of social work students…I was of course interested in this kind of training.[15]

The Beth Israel Hospital became a training center for medical and psychiatric social workers due to the early work of the Social Service Committee when Maida became its chair. In the Social Service Department's thirtieth anniversary celebration in 1958, Mrs. Martha Waldstein became the first designated psychiatric social worker at Beth Israel.

Maida, reflecting in her memoir on what the Social Service Department had achieved, quoted Martha Waldstein:

The general hospital offers a large reservoir of learning relevant to social work education, both in its generic and specific aspects. The school fieldwork unit can serve as an effective means of transmitting this knowledge to students. School supervisors could contribute to the improvement of field-work training by trying out combinations of learning experiences…by applying sound educational principles to these experiences, identifying the teaching points and arranging them in an orderly progression, school supervisors might develop a field-work course which would receive the same recognition from universities as the academic curriculum.

That's quite a statement and I believe it carries out some of…my thinking…about education and what I was trying to do at the school [Simmons], the material which I think is of interest to the development of psychiatric social work, and most relevant today.[16]

Notes to Chapter 4: Psychiatric Social Work

1 Oral Memoir, 2:239
2 Strean, Herbert S. "Applying Psychoanalytic Principles to Social Work Practice: An Historical Review," Edward and Sanville (eds.), *Fostering Healing and Growth, A Psychoanalytic Social Work Approach*, Jason Aronson, Inc., 1996, pp.2-3.
3 *The Encyclopedia of Social Work*, 16th ed., National Association of Social Workers. New York, 1971, 2:1239-1240.
4 Oral Memoir, 2:254-255
5 ibid., 2:262-264
6 ibid., 2:280
7 ibid., 2:282-283
8 Lunbeck, Elizabeth, *The Psychiatric Persuasion—Knowledge, Gender, and Power in Modern America*, (Princeton University Press) p.51.
9 ibid., 2:291-292
10 Maida Herman Solomon papers, MS 21, The Colonel Merriam E. Perry Archives, Simmons College, Boston, MA.
11 Oral Memoir, 2:306-308
12 ibid., 2:311
13 ibid., 2:312
14 ibid., 2:316-317
15 ibid., 2:318-319
16 ibid., 2:320-321

5
The Simmons Years

Of the many accomplishments in Maida's long and illustrious
career, one of the most significant was her work developing
and implementing curricula for a Master's Degree for the psychiatric social work sequence at the Simmons College School of Social
Work, where she began teaching in the fall of 1934. She was one of a
very small group of consummate social work professionals who not only
"invented" the field of psychiatric social work, but also oversaw its definition, its development of standards, and its integration with the other
institutions of modern American medicine and education—in short, its
professionalism. A colleague recounts, "Upon being asked if she
[Maida] was a graduate social worker, she replied that she was not—because she helped to write the first curriculum and the first examinations
and thus was excluded from officially taking either one."[1]

In an article in the Simmons College School of Social Work Alumni
Newsletter, Barbara Bryant, '50, reviewed the history of the school.
Describing the period in which Maida was active there, Bryant re-
ported:

> Miss Hardwick's tenure as Director of the School took her through the
> great depression and World War II, 1929-1952, and into the postwar
> years when our country became a global power and all things seemed
> possible...She attracted many distinguished teachers, including Harriett
> Bartlett in Medical Social Work, and Maida Solomon in Psychiatric So-
> cial Work...These individuals stayed with the School for many years
> and greatly influenced its direction.

Maida was recruited by Katherine Hardwick, with the mandate to
"beef up the mental health and psychiatric social work program at the

school."[2] The Encyclopedia of Social Work describes the institutional status of social work education just prior to and during the time of Maida's tenure:

> By 1932 a minimum curriculum had been adopted [by the American Association of Schools of Social Work (AASSW)]. In 1935 the AASSW had ruled that only those schools of social work which were established within an institution of higher learning on the approved list of the American Association of Universities were eligible for admission…
>
> By 1939 the Association had taken the further step of requiring as a condition of membership that schools of social work offer their educational programs on the graduate level, with the master's degree to be awarded upon completion of two years of graduate professional study…The National Council of Social Work Education (NCSWE) was established in 1946 to bring together representatives of the two associations [the AASSW and the National Association of Schools of Social Administration (NASSA)], the professional membership organizations, and the colleges and universities, to resolve the problems of educational standards. A 1951 study of social work education, undertaken by the National Council, contained proposals designed to resolve the issues. It led to the organization of the Council of Social Work Education (CSWE).[3]

The major emphasis of Maida's work was in the development and implementation of a curriculum for a two-year master's degree at Simmons. Toward that end, Maida developed psychiatric and mental health material so that the psychiatric social worker could take the knowledge gained in the classroom into the practice of the agency setting. She was also charged with the responsibility of providing psychiatric information for the medical information course at the school.

With the husband-wife team established at the Boston Psychopathic Hospital, Harry Solomon taught the clinical psychiatry course to Maida's second-year psychiatric social work students, developing a core curriculum around a syndrome. He introduced the patient interview into the classroom, enabling the student to witness first-hand the interaction between the psychiatrist and the patient. The clinical psychiatry course established in the late thirties continued with Dr. Solomon and later Dr. Elvin Semrad until the latter's death in 1976, and continued with others well into the 1980s.

Maida developed a course in human behavior for all second-year students at the school. The three earliest teachers were Drs. Bowman, Solomon, and Whitehorn, each of whom eventually became president of the American Psychiatric Association (APA). Other notable psychiatrists who taught at the school included Dr. Abraham Myerson, Dr. Grete Bibring, Dr. "Mo" Kaufman, Dr. Eveline Rexford, Dr. Avery Weisman, and Dr. Felix Deutch. The lecturers used the experience of teaching at Simmons to crystallize their ideas before writing them for publication.

Miss Hardwick gave Maida "free rein." While Miss Hardwick did not accept the heavily Freudian psychoanalytic approach, Maida later said, "She knew that I would present a well-rounded theoretical approach to students and in that way Hardwick could bear it."[4] In the early 1940s, Dr. Hans Sachs came from the Psychoanalytic Institute to teach the course on "The Psychoanalytic Theory of the Neurosis." Dr. Eleanor Pavenstadt also taught the same course later given by Dr. Elizabeth Zetzel, Maida's niece, Bess and Jim's daughter, who came to Boston after her husband's death in England. (Maida introduced Elizabeth to Dr. Lou Zetzel, whom she later married.) Maida described this period as being "highly analytic." Said she, "It was extremely difficult to combat the Viennese psychoanalytic influence."

The casework course and fieldwork practicum were an important part of the curriculum of the second-year program, advancing and augmenting the student's training from the first year and continuing to help the student integrate the teachings in the classroom with the practice of the fieldwork setting. [5]

The first-year casework course was taught by Miss Hardwick, whose tenure lasted until 1952. "She wanted her social workers to know everything about everything. She was not interested in specialization, but was very strong on poverty." Later, commented Maida, "Ethel Walsh, a very talented clinician and teacher, was brought to Simmons from the

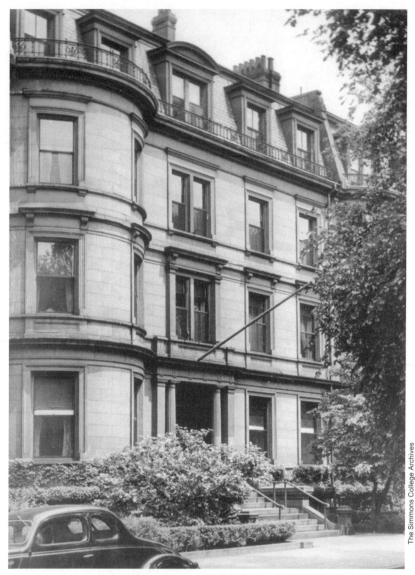

Simmons College School of Social Work
51 Commonwealth Avenue, Boston, Massachusetts, c. 1945.

Judge Baker Guidance Center. Walsh's approach to casework was much more psychoanalytic than Hardwick's."

Under Maida's leadership, Annette Garrett became the first teacher of the second-year casework course. She later taught at the Smith College School for Social Work. Louise Bandler was brought over from the Massachusetts General Hospital fieldwork unit to teach; she contributed a broad, practical, reality-based point of view and offered a nice balance to Walsh's narrower perspective.

In the first year the students spent two days in the field at placements. In the second year the students were in the field for three days a week. Academic work was crowded into two days. Second-year fieldwork units were established at the Beth Israel Hospital, the Boston State Hospital, and the Massachusetts General Hospital's Psychiatric Unit.

Both Ethel Cohen, chief of social work at Beth Israel, and Mrs. Martha Waldstein came to the school from the hospital, where they supervised a fieldwork training unit for the Simmons students. (Upon Maida's retirement from Simmons in 1957, Martha Waldstein assumed the direction of the psychiatric social work sequence.) Maida not only was given the administrative responsibilities for the psychiatric social work sequence, but also took full charge of teaching a four-credit directed-reading seminar to second-year students. As described in the Simmons College School of Social Work catalogue, it was designed to:

> …help the psychiatric social work student see psychiatric social work as part of the developing and changing fields of social work and psychiatry toward the ultimate goal of contributing both to preventive and curative mental health. The variations of field experience in psychiatric agencies afford in the classroom a blending of experience around the common core, which hopefully builds a point of view, moving from the specific and local to the more universal. Conversely, directed reading in the field of psychiatric social work and related areas should provide a broader background for current student field work and later practice, so that students may think in terms of the total mental health picture as well as specific psychiatric structural developments.

In one of the taped oral interviews with the author, Maida elaborated:

I hope that students acquire three things [from this course]: an orderly way of thinking about psychiatric social work with some historical perspective related to present day theory and practice of social work, etc.; some knowledge and understanding of the development and use of psychiatric agencies/units from the point of view of intra- and interprofessional relationships, etc.; some knowledge and understanding of the reasons for difficulties and limitations of psychiatric programs, etcetera.

Each student was required to keep a notebook of the activities at his or her fieldwork placement. These diaries were handed in to Maida four times a year and were vehicles that Maida and her associates would use in conferences with the students.

And it was not just the students of Simmons who felt the force of Maida's influence. In a recorded interview with Mr. Robert Rutherford, who assumed the position of director of the School of Social Work in 1952 (five years before Maida retired), he recalled,

As the wife of the then Superintendent of the Boston Psychopathic Hospital...she was able to provide a seemingly inexhaustible sequence of highly distinguished lecturers for the school. Other liaison with the community was achieved by Maida's volunteer service on a variety of community boards.

Mrs. Solomon was a model for her students as 'a career woman successfully juggling marriage, child rearing and career.' She shamelessly admits to putting pressure on students to devote some time to voluntary service and has tried to upgrade the concept and practice of volunteerism from the category 'into which people fit when they have nothing really to offer on a professional level.' A good portion of Mrs. Solomon's own work has been volunteered. At Simmons initially, she was paid for one day and worked four each week.

In her taped oral interview, Maida was asked about her effect on the school:

[I] did not think the academic world was 'quiet' then, any more than it is now... Dr. Richard Cabot was at the time an observer in Simmons faculty meetings. He was at times quite 'caustic'—[they were] lively meetings. Teachers defended what they taught. [I] may be responsible for making Simmons 'less and less quiet.' [I] went to Simmons to make changes and conflict was part of [my] life there and [I] flourished.

She would proudly declare:

[I] did change the school—I was brought in to do so—[my] associates and students changed the school too. Harry Solomon claimed that I 'acquired the school.' Teaching made me more conscious and aware of my professional responsibilities.

Naturally, relations with colleagues were not all sweetness and light. Maida stood up for her program, her students, and her vision of the profession and the education required for it. One divisive issue was oral examinations:

There was discussion of the broader issues; orders (or changes) made by the various directors of the school, etc. [There was also] faculty anger (not necessarily acknowledged) around the fact that [I] had so many students in [my] program whom [I] wanted to see through the oral exams and complete the course. [I] prepared for each individual oral. [This] took a great deal of time in the spring of each year, so that [I] could be fair to the students. Miss Hardwick liked the orals…Mr. Rutherford didn't like them. He decided (without consultation) to omit orals. Many issues were brought up to faculty meetings as *fait accomplis*. Orals were one of these.[6]

Change, however, went far beyond issues of particular curricular requirements and personal turf battles. This was the era of professionalization and standardization of academic disciplines throughout American universities. The kinds of changes Maida helped Simmons negotiate altered the basic nature of social work education in the United States.

One such change, after World War II, was the breakdown of gender distinctions in the way careers were conceived and the way educational institutions prepared people for them. The Simmons School of Social Work previously had affiliations with all-male institutions, but now it began to admit males directly. Maida recalled that "there were no overt [negative] feelings; however, some may have felt that men would immediately get the 'big jobs' of leadership right away. Men moved more easily into administrative jobs. The same is true today [1976]. The whole women's movement has made some changes in jobs, [but] men do move more quickly up the administrative ladder."7

The standardization of the field of social work forced the Simmons faculty to debate, and finally agree to, giving up the undergraduate year at Simmons College. Students received a graduate [MS] degree after one postgraduate year. Their senior year was [also] spent at the school of social work." As Maida recalled, "The issue wasn't decided on its merits by the faculty, but by the National [National Council of Social Work Educators]." This in turn raised the larger issue: "How far we would be

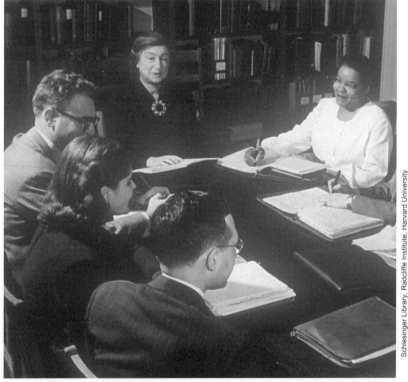

Maida Solomon teaching a class of graduate students, School of Social Work, Simmons College, c. 1955.

dominated, influenced, etc. by the national education group. They were having increasing influence—[their] concern [to standardize] the curriculum and accreditation. Simmons was accredited by being one of the early schools. Time came when they needed to be reaccredited. The faculty prepared 'violently' for accreditation." Miss Bartlett was very involved in National which she brought to faculty meetings regarding values, content, etc.

The professionalization and standardization of disciplines like social work benefited in large measure from the expansion of the federal government's funding for social programs during the Depression, the New Deal, and afterward, by means of agencies such as the Veterans Administration and the National Institute of Mental Health.

Part of Maida's energy was always channeled into finding funds for her students. She said:

[I] was interested in getting money for the training of psychiatric social workers. [My] first experience was through the AAPSW [American Association of Psychiatric Social Workers] to obtain scholarships through the Red Cross for students to work here and abroad, with the stipulation that the students work in that agency after completing their M.S. degree for a period of one to two years. Similarly for the army. This didn't work too well, as the workers wanted to be released from their commitment after graduation. Thus, they had to pay back the monies received if they didn't work at the Red Cross or Army after graduation. As a result, we dropped the programs.

We went to anyone for money—not really a scholarship, but perhaps 'bits of money'—$100 or so for books, etc. Jewish Women's Scholarships were one of the first organizations to give money. [I] wrote in the forties to every state in the union asking for money, i.e., New York, Pennsylvania, etc. [It was a] prolific way of getting students and money...

The federal government was the greatest source of funding. The VA was utilized as a [training] unit which also paid stipends. NIMH [National Institute of Mental Health] was a great resource. Simmons was one of the first schools to secure money to train students at such places as the BPH [Boston Psychopathic Hospital], Judge Baker, MGH-Psych Unit, etc. [I] found I had to influence the students to take placements which offered stipends…In the last few years [1950s], probably over one-half the students received some kind of financial aid.[8]

, One price of professionalization and standardization was the threat that people, the people whose distress had motivated Maida, her husband, her parents, the Hechts—the whole tradition of social service in which Maida stood—would get lost in the process; that they would become abstractions for social workers inculcated with increasingly formalized knowledge.

Maida would have none of it. To charges that social work education relied too much on practical "learning by doing" out in the field, that it was not an education but an "apprenticeship," she responded:

> We are definitely dependent upon an adequate experience in a good agency…one which offers good supervision, a learning caseload, a good relationship with other disciplines, particularly psychiatrists. But an 'apprenticeship'?[9]
>
> It's not close [she said] provided that supervision is offered from the school, and that we did! We selected agencies, supervisors, and met with them. There was a great deal of collaboration between the school and the agencies. The school offered a course for supervisors, taught by Miss Walsh. The question is more of whether or not supervisors in the field were close enough to the faculty. That is a continuing question. The students and the alumni association are now more in the picture [in 1976]. That poses a number of issues. [One needs] enough time in a given carefully selected agency to develop [oneself] as a student and to see what develops when you move on. [There is a] continual demand to integrate academic training with practice…today and twenty years ago.[10]

And Maida made sure that if practice informed theory, her students brought the best theory—rooted, in turn, in the best clinical practice—to their training. Often there were more visiting lecturers in her program than there were students. She tried to get the best people to teach a particular course, utilizing them for a greater or lesser time.

Robert Rutherford, MSW, former director of the Simmons College School of Social Work remarked:

I think one of Mrs. Solomon's great contributions was to provide all students with a firm, rich grounding in the best thinking practice in the mental health field...My introduction to mental illness came [as a student at the School of Social Work] at the Massachusetts Mental Health Center by Dr. Harry Solomon's interviewing patients. I was lucky enough to have had Dr. Grete Bibring teach my class in psychopathology.

One of our well-known psychiatrists told me, 'I learned my psychiatry from Harry Solomon and Elvin Semrad'...and I thought, 'So too did I,' and so too did other students at the School of Social Work...I am not an expert in the field, but I was well and truly and usefully indoctrinated. This, I think, is the great contribution Mrs. Solomon made, to provide excellence in presenting the best thinking from the fields of psychiatry and mental health, and insert this as an important building block in understanding the complexities of the people we are trying to help. If this understanding is in place, other things—administration, supervision, community work—can be added safely.[11]

Maida stated:

There was an issue of whether one was making the material real and lively for the students or creating confusion. Some students may not have 'been equal to' the number of lecturers. As time went on lecturers had to move from giving whole courses to a lecture or two as a result of increasing demands made upon their professional careers, i.e. one course was divided into four or five sections with several lecturers. What was missing in continuity was made up by excitement. The learning often provided questions which were taken up with fieldwork supervisors. By 1976 there probably were not the 'luminaries in the field' teaching at schools of social work; a younger group taught.[12]

Prominent in this "star-studded vaudeville show" (as Mr. Rutherford described) of social work academicians were, of course, the psychiatrists.

Said Maida:

I kept in touch with agencies; I knew what was going on...We often heard of a good person who would come and give a lecture. Also, a number of instructors and assistants in psychiatry at the Harvard Medical School were 'related' to Simmons social workers. Because of my husband's position at Harvard and Psycho he knew good speakers. When [I]

went to see people to [ask them to] come to Simmons, they knew that I
was related. This helped! Students also provided input as to good people
who might come.[13]

Robert Rutherford spoke thusly at Maida's memorial service:

But what did she do? Where was her imprint? Her mark? She carried
high in all places a banner on which was inscribed Psychiatric Social
Work. This was her cause, her motto, and her karma. Because of her efforts the social worker has a better, more secure, responsible position in
the treatment of mental and emotional illness—that social workers have
something useful, necessary, special to bring to the process of helping
people devastated by psychoses and neuroses, as well as a preventive
function social workers can assume. There is also a preparatory curriculum that equips workers to perform treatment functions as well—the establishment of that position and its educational program won largely,
almost entirely, by Maida Solomon. Although it were not enough to
have established a sub-profession, won its acceptance, created its curriculum—I recognize that she would never have called psychiatric social
work a 'sub' anything. For her it was a cut above. Her insistence on this
was as legendary as it was complete.[14]

The focus and continuity of Maida's career, from the Psycho through
the postwar Simmons years, gave her a sense of intellectual balance and
an ability to take the long view. Asked to comment on the issue that had
most vexed her field during her time at Simmons—the question of the
relative value of generic versus specific knowledge in social
work—Maida reflected, "The issue has been with us—it has gone
through cycles in [my teaching] lifetime—and continues to go through
cycles." She explained:

In the 1920s when [I] was president of the AAPSW, the Milford [Con-
necticut] conference took up the issue of generic versus specific. No one
knew what was generic and what was specific. A pamphlet [that came
out of the conference] was reprinted in 1974 or 1975. I thought there
was a large amount of material generic to the practice of social work.
There has also been specific material related to people with specific interests. The same is true sixty years later. During twenty-three years at
Simmons, [I] gave the generic as well as the specific material to psychiatric social workers in the second year.

86

The Simmons Years

There has been a battle which has raged over the years. The psychiatric social workers have become disliked because they had high standards of practice; they had an MS degree; [they] worked out what should be taught in schools and nationally through the National Association [NASW] and prior to that, the AAPSW.

The psychoanalytic movement which swept the country [when Maida started at the school] became extremely popular, and a great deal of analytic thinking was taught at the school. Social work agencies wanted to be called 'psychiatric.' Perhaps they risked too much. Perhaps they should have given greater validity to family problems by family agencies rather than to rush onto the psychiatric bandwagon.

As a result of increased social welfare, many agencies lost their reason for being [which] may be why they became so interested in the psychiatric area. In recent years the battle has changed. The psychoanalytic movement has suffered drawbacks. They have had to change their methodology, i.e., the number of times [per week] they see people, goals, etc. There is vituperation against psychiatry and psychiatrists. [I] don't think the battle has been lost, but must be researched to know its values. Basically, we must [continue to] develop good social work in education, research and mental health.[15]

Notes to Chapter 5: The Simmons Years

1 Comment by Dr. Miles F. Shore, former Superintendent, Massachusetts Mental Health Center.

2 Barbara Bryant, "Finding Our Educational Roots," Simmons School of Social Work, Alumni Newsletter, summer 1992.

3 *The Encyclopedia of Social Work*, NASW, 1971, 1:258-259.

4 Unless otherwise noted, the following quotations come from the authors' transcribed taped oral interviews of Maida Herman Solomon, December 7, 1976 to June 13, 1977, at Mrs. Solomon's home, 55 Lochstead Avenue, Jamaica Plain, MA, and are part of the archival collection at the Schlesinger Library, Radcliffe Institute, Harvard University.

5 Highlights of the Founding and First Seventy-Five Years of the Simmons School of Social Work (7/12/79), Simmons College Archives

6 From taped oral interviews

7 ibid.

8 ibid.

9 ibid.

10 ibid.

11 Robert Rutherford, MSW, Eulogy, March 30, 1988 for Maida H. Solomon, Massachusetts Mental Health Center.

12 from taped oral interviews

13 Oral Memoirs

14 Robert Rutherford, MSW, remarks at a memorial March 30, 1988 for Maida Herman Solomon, Massachusetts Mental Health Center.

15 ibid.

6

"Mrs. S"

The year 1957 was another major turning point in Maida's life. After twenty-three years of organizing, developing, and teaching the psychiatric social work sequence for second-year students at the Simmons College School of Social Work, she stepped down, receiving the title of Professor Emeritus of Social Economy. The twenty-three-year period of Maida's work came to a close not because of any loss of energy or infirmity, but because she was required by college regulations to retire at the age of sixty-six.

"I didn't want to leave at all," she said, "because I felt able to go on and [was] interested and had all kinds of plans and a study in progress. But I did learn from my husband that when you get through with something, you're through with it, and when the academic life is over you must accept that."[1] Consequently, in the following year, when she was asked by Mr. Rutherford to make a study of jobs and people, she decided not to, and the study was never made.

Among the many tributes and honors bestowed upon Maida at her retirement was the annual Maida H. Solomon Award. This was established by the students, alumni, and faculty of the school for outstanding research carried out by a psychiatric social work graduate from the Simmons College School of Social Work.

Mary Breslin, MSW, recalled driving Maida home from an awards committee meeting one night:

> I think we met at Harriett Bartlett's home in Cambridge. [Ms. Bartlett chaired the department of medical social work and an award was named in her honor.] Anyway, I was working at St. Margaret's at the time and so I was assigned by the committee to work with the Bartlett group.

This didn't please me too much but so it was. It didn't please Maida either. She certainly considered me one of "her girls". On the way to Jamaica Plain I was questioned about working in a medical setting where the patients were essentially physically healthy but presented with major psychosocial issues/problems. It was not an easy task. It was quite a conversation, I can assure you. The interesting thing about that job, by the way, was that my department [Mary was then the director of the department of social services at the hospital] was the only full-time mental health component in the hospital. And we were used as such!

For many years Maida served as a member of the awards committee, reviewing articles by her former students as well as by recent Simmons School of Social Work graduates. This award has been given annually since 1957.

Harry, then superintendent of the Massachusetts Mental Health Center, as well as Bullard Professor of Psychiatry at the Harvard Medical School, was very interested in his wife's plans upon her retirement from Simmons. He felt that Maida should continue to contribute her special talents as a teacher and researcher. He voiced his opinion to

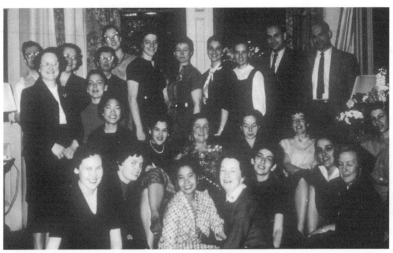

Maida (middle, center row), at her retirement party sponsored by Class of 1957, Simmons College School of Social Work, 1957.

Dr. Milton Greenblatt, then his Assistant Superintendent and Director of Clinical Research. Dr. Greenblatt was pleased to invite Maida to become involved in the increasingly busy and productive Social Research department.

The Community Mental Health Act, passed by Congress in 1954, created federal funding for many studies. During this time psychotropic medications were being developed and coming into increasing usage in state hospitals. State and private monies were also available to researchers to study alternatives to hospitalization as well as the efficacy of various medications for the mentally ill and emotionally disturbed. Several new proposals had been funded, with psychiatric social workers included.

Carrying over her lifelong interest in research, Maida accepted Dr. Greenblatt's invitation. Dr. Greenblatt created an unfunded position for Maida as Consultant in Social Psychiatry and Social Work Research.

Joan Morse, MSW (a daughter of Judge Abraham E. Pinanski, one of several men Maida saw socially after graduating from Smith College) recalled:

> I worked for five years at the Massachusetts General Hospital in neurology, married and had four children. I really came to know MHS [Maida Herman Solomon] when my children were in school and I was ready to return to work. She had just retired from Simmons but remained retired for only a few days. She then [helped to] set up a unit at the Massachusetts Mental Health Center for clinical research, employing married social workers with children who wanted to work part-time.
>
> My own assignment was an NIH [National Institutes of Health] funded study of the comparative value of psychotherapy and medication in a double-blind study of schizophrenic young men.
>
> She introduced me to research design, screening patients from several state hospitals, interviewing parents, and the first year of a treatment program...I was grateful to MHS...she was a practical constructive guide in an atmosphere very psychoanalytical at the time.

The author, a June 1957 graduate of the psychiatric social work program at Simmons, had been hired right out of school into a newly funded National Institute of Mental Health research grant.

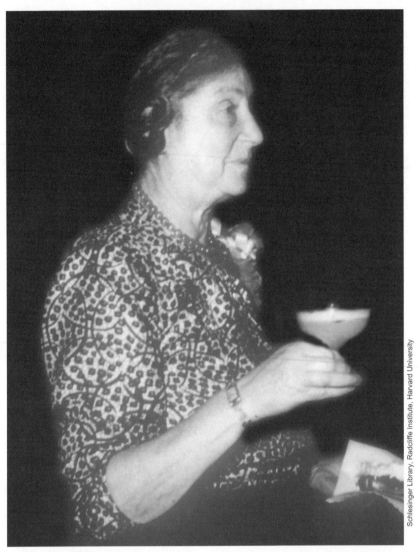

Maida Solomon at a party given in her honor by the Class of 1957 upon her retirement from teaching, Simmons College, 1957.

Like a number of other recent graduates, I had only limited experience for the job: two courses in research, one course in statistics, and a jointly authored thesis. Although interviewing the families of the patients included in the study,[2] for which we had been trained—in the classroom and in supervised fieldwork—the formulation, gathering of data, and writing were areas in which I was less confident.

The appearance of "Mrs. S," as we called her, made an enormously positive impact on all of us fledgling researchers. She was able to shore us up whenever we were weak. She held us to high standards while making it possible for us to attain something like those expectations.

Eva Deykin, PhD (a fellow social worker on the "Drug and Social Therapies" project) recalled:

I remember vividly going over with Mrs. Solomon a paper I had written and was expecting to submit for publication. She insisted that it needed rewriting despite my naïve view that it was just fine. We worked over each sentence with Mrs. Solomon hunting for exactly the right words that would convey the precise nuance of intended meaning. She searched for the words in the same way a master craftsman jeweler sifts through a collection of stones to find the one whose shape, color and size is perfect for the overall design.

It was painstaking work but the finished product was clearly superior. I learned a great deal that cold winter afternoon as the pallid sun shone through the window of her small cluttered office. I understood then that excellence does not just happen; it must be pursued with hard work and a constant critical approach.

Throughout her career, Maida also was able to help many young, trained, professional social workers to combine careers with marriage and children. She was instrumental in creating part-time employment opportunities for a large number of women who wanted to pursue their personal and professional interests.

Maida was famous for her up-to-date card file she kept on the status of each one of her students. A few years after a student left work to begin a family she was likely to receive a phone call from Maida asking, "Well, isn't it time you came to work again," mentioning a position she had already lined up.

Mollie Grob, MSW recalled:

She [Maida Herman Solomon] reached me when I was fully occupied raising three young children with the suggestion that I 'get out of the kitchen.' This resulted in my return to work in a fully satisfying and meaningful career in the mental health field.

A few years later when I had the opportunity to redirect my psychiatric skills from clinical practice to outcome research with psychiatric patients and their families, I made the transition—following the model she inspired.

We met regularly in her later years when I became a member of the Simmons Alumni Awards Committee over which she presided. Then I found it rewarding to observe her gratification and significance to the mental health community.

During her post-retirement period, Maida expanded her career as a research consultant from the Massachusetts Mental Health Center to the Boston State Hospital (Milton Greenblatt brought Maida and a number of us social work researchers to the Boston State Hospital in 1965 when he assumed the position of its Superintendent), the Metropolitan State Hospital and the Rutland Corner Halfway House, in which she took a special interest, to name a few.

At the Boston State Hospital several psychiatric social work researchers had the benefit of Maida Solomon's expertise.

Margaret (Peg) Goldberg, MSW remembered Maida thusly:

I knew and worked with Maida Herman Solomon [The Volunteer Case Aide Program and the Massachusetts Academy of Psychiatric Social Work] for many years...I always felt her warmth and intelligence. She was tough and demanding but fair and helpful—a great teacher. She possessed wit and a large sense of humor, and was fun to be with. I learned a great deal from her and always felt her support...she was an extraordinary woman who inspired respect and affection in me. As I remember her, a smile comes to my face.

Shirley Jacobson, MSW shared her feelings toward and experience of Maida:

Personally, her impact was of tremendous significance. After my first child was born...she contacted me about a research project—a study of in-patient depressed women funded by the NIMH [at the Boston State Hospital.] It was a four hour per week position doing combined clinical

94

"Mrs. S"

and research with families of women. I had not planned to be a working mother and had serious doubts. MHS helped me to make the initial decision…she had a most effective ability to see the long-range issues, i.e., when negotiation for funding or a salary, etc., to always aim high—ask for more than you expect or hope to receive. Due to her example she showed me how to be strong, but humane, caring and empathic. I continued to work in the area of research and was later encouraged by her to return to Simmons, to become 'legitimate'…to get my MSW. She gave me courage to take all that on, to write and ultimately publish.

Perhaps Dr. Milton Greenblatt summed up Maida's enormous skills and energy best, describing her as a "thinker-upper," a "worker-througher," and a "getter-doner."

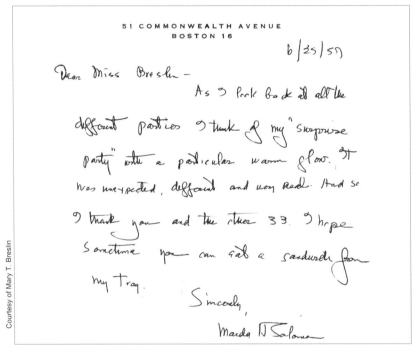

Thank-you note from Maida Solomon to Mary T. Breslin
for silver tray given to Maida by the Class of 1957.

In talking about her retirement, Maida said:

My time went down from forty-five to fifty hours a week [at Simmons] to twenty to thirty hours a week…it varied depending on what I was doing at any particular time…of course my husband [had] retired and we spent a lot more time together and I would say we took on more traveling.[3]

According to son Eric:

Harry Solomon actually retired at age seventy-nine, and at eighty-one returned to work part-time at the Bedford VA Hospital, becoming full-time Acting Director at eighty-three before final retirement at eighty-five. Thus it was appropriate for Maida to work through her eighties.

Several people interviewed Maida for archival collections: Eva Moseley, archivist at the Schlesinger Library; Barbara Miller Solomon, a dean at Harvard as well as daughter-in-law to Maida and Harry; Elizabeth Gould Herrera and myself, both of us psychiatric social work researchers and graduates of Simmons College School of Social Work during Maida's tenure at the school.

During one interview, Ms. Herrera interrupted her questions with a "personal" recollection:

As a student of yours in the middle 1950s, subsequently with my placement at Psycho [and later as a researcher at the Rutland Corner House], I remember the dominant themes of Mrs. Solomon…Those were excellence of performance…getting [material] down on paper, evaluating work in a structured, competent research way, writing for the record and maintaining a very high level of professional integrity in all work that was done…

The other thing I might say is that, unlike some consultants…Mrs. S stayed extremely active [and] made many helpful suggestions and didn't just [allow] something to pass over a desk and go without many revisions and suggestions.

Family members recalled that during the "retirement" years, Mrs. S. remained very interested in and attentive to her former students and colleagues, and continued her professional activities at home. Concerned about those who had labored for her at home, Mrs. S. worked hard to get appropriate housing and full Social Security benefits for one of her long-time household employees, Mrs. Wright. Maida, herself then well into her eighties, visited Mrs. Wright once a week until the latter's death in her nineties. Maida encouraged other Solomon family members to also visit her.

Maida became engaged in another kind of activity in the late 1960s and early 1970s. While at the Boston State Hospital in 1969-1970, Eleanor Gay, then chief of the Department of Psychiatric Social Work, met with Maida to discuss the possibility of forming a new professional organization of trained and experienced psychiatric social workers who would come together "to further the practice and research activities of psychiatric social work; to further the interests, maintain and advance the standards of practice; to advance education directed toward the improvement of social work skills and to make available such knowledge for increasing skills in clinical practice."[4]

In May 1971 the Massachusetts Academy of Psychiatric Social Work (recently renamed the Massachusetts Society of Clinical Social Work) was incorporated in the Commonwealth of Massachusetts. Throughout its conception, birth, and development as the organization we now know, Maida Solomon's imprimatur was clearly evident. Her creativity, productivity, and wise counsel all left their mark.

In a statement prepared and read by Maida at an academy dinner on October 20, 1976, she recalled:

> I remember seven or eight years ago seriously discussing with this same person how and when an Academy of Psychiatric Social Work could be formed to further service, education and community relationships toward the goal of better mental health of the mentally ill and emotionally disturbed. You in 1975 and 1976 are that professional group and this person was then our President, Eleanor Gay [who served as the Academy's first President from 1971-1975] for whom the Directors and Executive Committee were pleased to create the annual Eleanor Gay Lecture of the Massachusetts Academy of Psychiatric Social Work as an integral part of the Academy's social work program.[5]

What was not said was that Maida herself had been essential in the planning and creation of the organization that had been so well realized. She was later honored by an annual lecture at the Academy given in her name.

Indeed many honors and accolades came to her. On February 21, 1979, Jill Conway, President of Smith College, presented the Smith College Medal Award to Maida H. Solomon, Class of 1912:

> Educator, researcher, leader in the establishment of the mental health professions, pioneer in study of the problems of adolescence and of depression in women. To recount the significant points on your career is to describe the establishment of your profession. You were a pioneer when you began working at Boston Psychopathic Hospital in 1916 and you have remained one all your life. In 1934, you began your formal academic career as a faculty member at the Simmons College School of Social Work, and during your twenty-three years at that distinguished

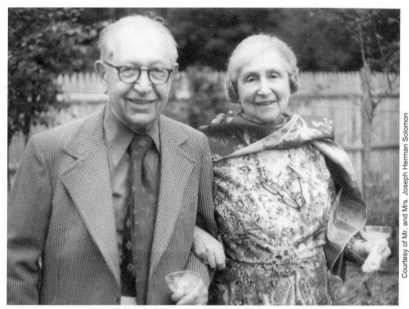

Courtesy of Mr. and Mrs. Joseph Herman Solomon

Partners: Dr. Harry C. Solomon and Maida Herman Solomon, at their sixtieth wedding anniversay celebration, June 27, 1976.

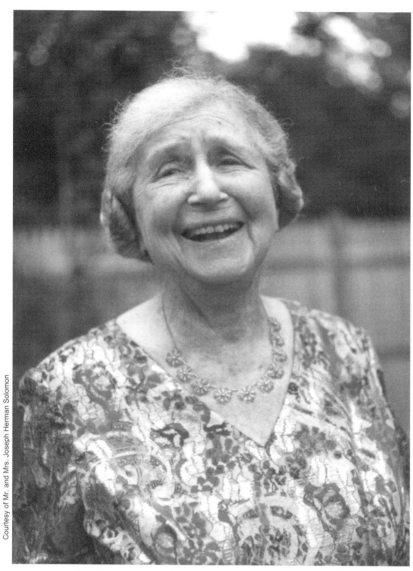

Maida Herman Solomon, age 85, at her sixtieth
wedding anniversay celebration.

school, you gave your passion for research, your professional standards
and your talents as a clinician to hundreds of students. You have never
retired from the calling of the scientist, and your capacity for encouraging others to take a scientific approach to unsolved problems in human
behavior has made you one of the most effective leaders in research in
the mental health field. Your sense of your calling made you one of the
founders of the American Association of Psychiatric Social Work [now
the National Association of Social Workers] and one of the key figures
in setting standards for your profession. Your twenty-eight publications
have ranged from your early work on the disturbed adolescent to studies
on the alternatives to hospitals in mental health care. All have been informed by your unquenchable curiosity and your vision of human dignity. We are proud to celebrate your long and fruitful career and to
award you a Smith College Medal.

In a profile of "Grande Dames" in *Boston Magazine*, December 1979,
Maida was described as a vibrant personality:

A pioneer in the field of psychiatric social work, and a former department head at the Simmons School of Social Work, Maida Herman Solomon remains so active she needs three desks in her home in Jamaica
Plain. 'I am retired only from Simmons, not my profession,' she reminds
the reporter, before ticking off a long list of current projects. These include consulting to mental health centers and holding civic and professional board memberships.

At eighty-eight, Solomon still enjoys swimming and playing tennis on
her own court. But ask for her health secrets and she proffers a dish of
chocolate mints. 'I love candy,' she says enthusiastically. 'I never smoke
much...only three cigarettes a day now, and I have an occasional cock-
tail'. She does note that she is hearty. 'I don't catch colds easily and if I
do, I become outraged,' she says laughing.

In a recent speech to many of her colleagues, Solomon summed up her
lifelong efforts to bring about social change: 'In 1915 I carried a visible
banner for women's suffrage on Boylston Street in Boston. Now in
1979, I carry an invisible banner for all of you who are pioneering in psychiatric social work.'[6]

Maida was "inducted" into the National Academy of Practice in
1982. Founded in 1981 to advise governmental bodies on the problems
of health care, the NAP was "dedicated to serving as the nation's distin-

guished forum that addresses and promotes education, research and
public policy related to improving the quality of health for all through
interdisciplinary care…Distinguished practitioners are individuals who
have spent a significant portion of their professional career as practitioners in the direct delivery to, and practice of health care to the con-
sumer; Distinguished Scholars are elected for their academic careers;
both are judged by the Academy to which they retain to have made significant and enduring contributions."

There are ten academies that include, among others, the disciplines
of medicine, social work, nursing, and psychology. Each of the academies is limited to 150 Active Distinguished Practitioners or Scholars in
their respective fields.[7]

A second prestigious honor was awarded to Maida, this time by the
Smith College School for Social Work. On July 25, 1987, the Day-
Garrett Award was presented to her by Kenneth H. McCartney, Acting
President of Smith College:

> Maida Herman Solomon—by building on the training offered you at
> Smith College, you have become a renowned educator, researcher,
> leader in the establishment of the mental health professions, and pioneer
> in the study of the problems of adolescence and of depression in women.
> Your pioneer role began at Boston Psychopathic Hospital in 1916 and
> has continued ever since. In your twenty-three years as a faculty mem-
> ber at the Simmons College School of Social Work, you inspired count-
> less students with your passion for research, your high professional
> standards and your talents as a clinician. Your twenty-eight publications,
> ranging from early work on disturbed adolescents to studies on the alter-
> natives to hospitals in mental health care, amount to a body of scientific
> contributions of remarkable scope and leadership in research in the
> mental health field. Your founding role in the American Association of
> Psychiatric Social Workers [now the National Association of Social
> Workers] attests to your sense of calling in the social work profession.
>
>   Smith College was proud to celebrate your distinguished career with
> the award of a Smith College Medal in 1979. Tonight we are proud to
> celebrate your outstanding professional career and to award you the
> Day-Garrett Award.

In 1979, Milton Greenblatt, MD (Maida's former "boss" at the Psycho), described Maida thusly:

> I cannot possibly detail the myriad of ways in which Mrs. Solomon helped me personally as a fledgling research director, and later State Hospital Superintendent [Boston State Hospital] over a period of years. She is the most progressive, positive and entrepreneurial person I have known. This, besides her gifts as a social worker, teacher, and collaborator with her husband on much earlier works, such as *Syphilis of the Innocent* which is regarded as a classic in its field. Eternally youthful in spirit and outlook, always the student learning and growing, magnificent teacher, mentor to many hundreds of young professionals, and mature intellectuals—I have not seen her peer in my lifetime, and of course I never expect to have anyone make so generous a contribution to my career as did Mrs. Solomon. This [is] purely a personal reflection. Her contribution to her own professional field and to the mentally ill generally stands enduring above all."[8]

Harry Solomon passed away at the age of ninety-two on May 23, 1982, but Maida continued to celebrate life until January 25, 1988, when she died at ninety-six years of age.

Notes to Chapter 6: "Mrs. S"

1 Oral Memoir, 3:574-575.
2 Greenblatt, M. Solomon, H; Evans, A.S. and Brooks, G. (eds.), *Drugs and Social Therapies in Chronic Schizophrenia*, Charles Thomas, Springfield, IL. 1965.
3 ibid., 3:575-577.
4 Massachusetts Academy of Psychiatric Social Work, Articles of Incorporation, 1971.
5 Speech delivered at the Massachusetts Academy of Psychiatric Social Work dinner meeting creating the Eleanor Gay Annual Lecture, October 20, 1976.
6 *Boston Magazine* 71, no. 12 (December 1979) p.134.
7 The National Academies of Practice, Background Information, Nicholas A. Cumming, PhD, ScD, Founding President, 2001
8 From a letter written by Dr. Milton Greenblatt, July 18, 1979 to Mrs. Susan Bailis; Chairman, Simmons College School of Social Work, Awards Committee.

Afterword

There is a measure of sadness as we join in these moments of tribute and farewell to Maida, who was a major influence in our lives. Students in the hundreds were beneficiaries of her passion for excellence, and I have met women social workers who spoke of her with unbounded admiration and awe; but we family members and friends were special recipients of her concern, her guidance, and her love, and we shall miss her colorful presence. Life won't be quite the

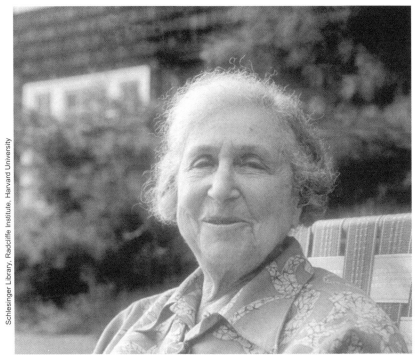

At home, enjoying Harry's garden, Jamaica Plain, MA, c. 1979.

same, now that Maida Solomon has, at a wonderful age, been called from this world.

Our sadness is tempered, perhaps, by the knowledge of her very many years; I don't recall ever conducting a funeral service for anyone much older than she...Indeed, though parting be sad, our mood might well be one of rejoicing; of rejoicing in the fact that Maida lived, and was so important a part of our lives; of rejoicing in her many professional accomplishments; and especially, of rejoicing because Maida herself felt pleased with the life she had lived. A few years ago, before Harry died, and in anticipation of death, she wrote, in a note to Joe, "The intent of this letter is to say we've had a great time together on this earth, with all our kids, their spouses, their kids and their spouses." [Had she written this a little later, she would certainly have added a word about the great-grandchildren, who totaled an impressive eleven in number.] How wonderful that someone nearing life's end could write so enthusiastically. Perhaps it was the evident disparity between her own favored situation and the problems borne by so much of humanity that prompted her to devote her energies, in such large measure, to the welfare of fellow people. "Loneliness kills" was printed on the bumper sticker of her car, and Maida meant it and tried all her life to do something about it.

Maida had an outstanding career as a researcher, author and professor at Simmons College, about which I know only what I have read in her curriculum vitae, and about which I shall not speak, except to mention that there are archives of her scholarly material at Simmons and Radcliffe; and to add some of the phrases spoken to her when, in 1979, at the age of eighty-seven, she was awarded a Smith College Medal (and incidentally, Maida just last Spring [1987], marched, amazingly, at her 75th class reunion at Smith.)

"You were a pioneer [the citation read] when you began working at the Boston Psychopathic Hospital in 1916 and you have remained one all your life. You gave your passion for research, your professional standards and your talents as a clinician to hundreds of students." She was called one of the most effective leaders in research in the mental health field, and "one of the key figures in setting standards in her profession." Finally she was saluted for her unquenchable curiosity and her vision of human dignity. Maida as we know, received many other honors, and the American Jewish Committee has made a 650-page oral history of her life. She was a high achiever, a role model to many, and she always held herself—and others—to the highest standards. She kept in touch with many former students, and was thus an ongoing important figure in their lives and their careers.

It was as a family friend that I knew Maida, whom, when I was a child, I of course called "Aunt Maida," in the style of those long-ago days. You knew it when she entered a room, or when she was merely in a room and you knew she was a special person. She dressed as she chose, not as current style dictated. She spoke her mind freely and frankly, perhaps sometimes a little too frankly, commenting, for example, on a few unwanted pounds that I might have put on, or on a particularly clumsy tennis shot. She lived with flair and with verve, and in so doing was the perfect complement and life companion for Harry, who tended to be the quiet one, who looked on with wise understanding and with admiring heart. They traveled much together, each with a special personal sense of humor.

Maida had been educated in the classic manner. She had become an avid reader, and was a reader virtually all her life; she knew Latin and French, and English grammar, and sometimes let you know it. She loved tennis and swimming. Religiously, once a year she would drive an hour or more to come from Long Lake in Maine to our family's cottage on Birch Island, in Casco Bay. Once on the island she would take a brief swim, visit politely, and soon be on her return trip, mission accomplished. She adored her family's vacation properties in Maine, where the large Solomon clan knew togetherness. But with Maida in charge, of course, the togetherness was somewhat regulated. Maida would often orchestrate the comings and goings of various branches of the family; and once there, there were definite limitations of time and space. Each group was entitled to its private time and private place, just as she and Harry once were. Even her beloved trees were entitled to security of life and limb, and were not to be disturbed by human intrusion. If a tree is in the way, she said, then build the cabin somewhere else.

Maida would acquire what she wanted, and didn't care about wasting time doing things she really didn't care about, such as going shopping as a recreational activity. Nor did she use things just because they were stylish; I'm thinking of a little piece of plain white paper on which she so often wrote notes, and of the U.S. government stamped envelopes, with plain return address imprint, that was the hallmark of her correspondence. Maybe, somewhere, she had some proper elegant stationery—but I, for one, never saw it.

And maybe, although it's hard to imagine, maybe once in a long time Maida saw herself overruled—but I don't recall that ever happening. She was a determined person, who expected that what she wanted done would be done. In another note to Joe she described exactly what she wanted, and then added, "If any of this makes anyone unhappy, deal with it." (Which meant, of course, that her wishes were not to be changed.)

Maida, as we know, was not formally religious, but she was very conscious of the fact that she was Jewish, and had done her share for various Jewish organizations. But it is clear to me that the direction of her life, and the motivation for it, were thoroughly Jewish: the drive to "choose life," to make the most of herself and her years; the urgency to make a mark on society, so that she left the world better than she found it; her respect for God's world, and for all that lived and grew in it. She would, of course, have scoffed at the thought that she was the quintessential Jewish mother, but in some ways, she really was. As the familiar works in the Book of Proverbs put it:

> The heart of her husband doth safely trust in her; she doeth in him good and not evil all the days of her life; she considereth the field, and buyeth it; she stretcheth out her hand to the poor; strength and dignity are her clothing, and she laugheth at the time to come. She openeth her mouth with wisdom, and the law of kindness is on her tongue. Her children rise up and call her blessed; her husband also, and he praiseth her: many daughters have done valiantly, but thou excellest them all.

Afterword

Maida's son-in-law, Eph Radner, suggested to me that Maida's life might well be characterized by the word "constancy." There was constancy in her personal relationships: when she spoke with you, she also listened to what you had to say. If she was your friend—and Maida was blessed with good friends—she was your true friend, your constant friend. She was constant in her devotion to her favorite sports, constant in her vision of her profession, constant in her hope for a better world.

If that world ever comes, it will be partly because Maida Solomon had a hand in it. She was a remarkable, unforgettable woman, who took to heart the injunction of Ecclesiastes: "Whatsoever thy had findeth for thee to do, that do with all thy might."

Maida came into this world, and she lived with all her might. And that was good. Yes, dear friends, it was *Tov M'od*, it was very good. *Zecher tzaddik livracha*—The memory of the righteous is for an eternal blessing. Amen.

Rabbi H. Bruce Ehrmann

Author's note: Rabbi Ehrmann had a unique perspective of Maida and Harry, as the Solomons enjoyed a very close relationship with his parents, Sarah and Herbert Ehrmann. Rabbi Ehrmann granted the author permission to include this eulogy he gave at a private memorial service for Maida in 1988.

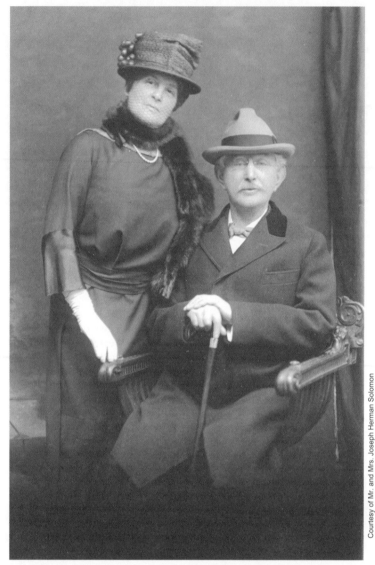

Courtesy of Mr. and Mrs. Joseph Herman Solomon

Maida Herman's parents, Joseph and Hennie Herman,
taken at Atlantic City, NJ, date unknown.

Maida Herman's Ancestors

Maida's Parents

Maida's father, Joseph Michael HERMAN, was born on 3 Apr 1851 in Altenkunstadt, Germany (Bavaria). He died on 9 Dec 1920 in Atlantic City, NJ. He was buried in Adath Israel Cemetery, Wakefield, MA. He married Hannah (Hennie) ADLER on 2 Nov 1881.

Maida's mother, Hannah (Hennie) ADLER, was born on 16 Nov 1862 in Baltimore, MD. She died on 25 Aug 1950 in Boston, MA. She was buried in Adath Israel Cemetery, Wakefield, MA.

Maida's grandparents

Maida's paternal grandfather, Michael HERRMANN, was born on 8 May 1814 in Altenkunstadt, Germany. He died on 21 Apr 1893 in Altenkunstadt, Germany. He was buried on 23 Apr 1893 in Burgkunstadt, Germany. He married Karoline (Gutel) BAUER in 1845.

Maida's paternal grandmother, Karoline (Gutel) BAUER, was born on 24 May 1822 in Ermreuth, Germany. She died on 27 May 1901 in Altenkunstadt, Germany. She was buried in Burgkunstadt, Germany.

Maida's maternal grandfather, Abraham Simon ADLER, was born on 12 Apr 1831 in Hofgeismar, Germany (Hesse). He died on 22 Jul 1915 in Baltimore, MD. He was buried in Baltimore Hebrew Congregation Cemetery. He married Sarah FRANK about 1860 in Baltimore, MD.

Maida's maternal grandmother, Sarah FRANK, was born on 27 Nov 1841 in Baltimore, MD. She died on 1 Dec 1864 in Baltimore, MD. She was buried in Baltimore Hebrew Congregation Cemetery.

Maida's great-grandparents

Maida's paternal great-grandfather, Salomon Josef HERRMANN, was born in 1777 in Altenkunstadt, Germany. He died on 13 Oct 1836 in Altenkunstadt, Germany. He was buried in Burgkunstadt, Germany. He married Mathilde (Magdalena) OPPENHEIMER in 1800.

Maida's paternal great-grandmother, Mathilde (Magdalena) OPPENHEIMER, was born on 3 Feb 1781 in Burgkunstadt, Germany. She died on 24 Jan 1854 in Altenkunstadt, Germany. She was buried in Burgkunstadt, Germany.

Maida's paternal great-grandfather, Moses Samuel BAUER, was born in 1786 in Ermreuth, Germany. He died on 26 Jan 1852 in Ermreuth, Germany. He married Sara SPATZ in 1805.

Maida's paternal great-grandmother, Sara SPATZ, was born in 1787 or 1788. She died on 29 May 1848 in Ermreuth, Germany.

Maida's maternal great-grandfather, Siemon Suessmann ADLER, was born on 12 Jul 1785 in Hofgeismar, Germany. (Death records unavailable.) He married Hannah STEINBERG.

Maida's maternal great-grandmother, Hannah STEINBERG, was born in 1790. (Death records unavailable.)

Maida's maternal great-grandfather, Simon FRANK, was born on 15 Oct 1807 in Kleinostheim, Germany (Bavaria). He died on 28 Jul 1869 in Baltimore, MD. He was buried in Baltimore Hebrew Congregation Cemetery. He married Fratel (Fanny) NAUMBURG in Mar 1841 in Baltimore, MD.

Maida's maternal great-grandmother, Fratel (Fanny) NAUMBURG, was born on 21 Apr 1816 in Treuchtlingen, Germany. She died on 25 Oct 1888 in Baltimore, MD. She was buried in Baltimore Hebrew Congregation Cemetery.

Maida Herman's Descendants

1. Maida HERMAN was born on 9 Mar 1891 in Boston, MA. She died on 25 Jan 1988 in Boston, MA. She was buried in Boston, MA. Maida married Harry Caesar SOLOMON on 27 Jun 1916 in Boston, MA. Harry was born on 25 Oct 1889 in Hastings, NE. He died on 23 May 1982 in Boston, MA. He was buried in Boston, MA. They had four children.

Maida and Harry's children

2. Peter Herman SOLOMON (Maida) was born on 6 Sep 1918 in Lynn, MA. He died on 24 Jun 1988 in Cambridge, MA. He was buried in Cambridge, MA (Mt. Auburn Cemetery). Peter married Barbara Leah MILLER on 13 May 1940 in New York City, NY. Barbara was born on 12 Feb 1919 in Boston, MA. She died on 24 Aug 1992 in Cambridge, MA. She was buried in Cambridge, MA (Mt. Auburn Cemetery). They had three children:
   + 6 Peter Herman SOLOMON Jr. was born on 24 Aug 1942.
   + 7 Maida Elizabeth SOLOMON was born on 8 Mar 1946.
   + 8 Daniel Miller SOLOMON was born on 5 Apr 1950.

3. Joseph Herman SOLOMON (Maida) was born on 23 Oct 1921 in Boston, MA. Joseph married Carolyn Krouse HELDMAN on 19 May 1945 in Cincinnati, OH. Carolyn was born on 9 May 1923 in Cincinnati, OH. They had three children:
   + 9 Jody Louise SOLOMON was born on 27 Mar 1947.
   + 10 Katherine Heldman SOLOMON was born on 30 Jul 1950.
   + 11 David Heldman SOLOMON was born on 25 Apr 1954.

4. Babette SOLOMON (Maida) was born on 9 Oct 1924 in Boston, MA. Babette married Ephraim RADNER on 4 Jun 1950 in Boston, MA.

Ephraim was born on 23 Oct 1921 in Springfield, MA. They had four children:

   12 Judith May RADNER was born on 28 Jul 1953 in Boston, MA.

   + 13 James Mark RADNER was born on 30 Aug 1955.

   14 Nancy Lee RADNER was born on 7 May 1957 in Boston, MA.

   + 15 Wendy Herman RADNER was born on 7 May 1957.

   5. H. Eric SOLOMON (Maida) was born on 8 Oct 1928 in Boston, MA. H. Eric SOLOMON married Irene Frances LEIDER on 1 May 1954 in New York City, NY. Irene was born on 8 Oct 1932 in New York City, NY. They had two children:

   + 16 Madeline Andrea SOLOMON was born on 9 May 1960.

   + 17 William Daniel SOLOMON was born on 13 Mar 1964.

Maida and Harry's grandchildren

   6. Peter Herman SOLOMON Jr. (Peter Herman SOLOMON, Maida) was born on 24 Aug 1942 in Boston, MA. Peter married Susan GROSS on 30 Jan 1965 in Montreal, Canada. Susan was born on 16 Apr 1943 in Montreal, Canada. They had the following children:

   18 Raphael SOLOMON was born on 8 Dec 1974 in Toronto, Canada.

   19 Rachel SOLOMON was born on 20 Apr 1977 in Toronto, Canada.

   7. Maida Elizabeth SOLOMON (Peter Herman SOLOMON, Maida) was born on 8 Mar 1946 in Boston, MA. Maida married Christopher ST. JOHN . THEY HAD THE FOLLOWING CHILD:

   + 20 Keisha SANCHEZ was born on 10 May 1975.

   8. Daniel Miller SOLOMON (Peter Herman SOLOMON, Maida) was born on 5 Apr 1950 in Boston, MA. Daniel married Diane Amy BLITSTEIN on 25 Nov 1984 in Oceanside, NY. Diane was born on 21 Jul 1953 in Brooklyn, NY. They had the following children:

   21 Zachary William SOLOMON was born on 21 Oct 1988 in Boston, MA. He died on 30 May 1998 in Coral Springs, FL.

22 Joshua Benjamin SOLOMON was born on 25 Aug 1992 in Boston, MA.

9. Jody Louise SOLOMON (Joseph Herman SOLOMON, Maida) was born on 27 Mar 1947 in Boston, MA. Jody married James Mark HORVITZ on 13 Aug 1972 in Newton, MA. James was born on 24 Dec 1946 in New Bedford, MA. They had the following children:

23 Lisa Kim HORVITZ was born on 4 Apr 1975 in Athens, OH.

24 Andrea Beth HORVITZ was born on 5 Oct 1977 in Newton, MA.

10. Katherine Heldman SOLOMON (Joseph Herman SOLOMON, Maida) was born on 30 Jul 1950 in Boston, MA. Katherine married Joseph Michael WOODWARD on 1 Jul 1973 in Newton, MA. Joseph was born on 21 Aug 1950 in Chicago, IL. They had the following children:

25 Andrew Solomon WOODWARD was born on 6 Apr 1982 in Washington, DC.

26 Pamela Gwendolyn WOODWARD was born on 3 Jun 1985 in Washington, DC.

11. David Heldman SOLOMON (Joseph Herman SOLOMON, Maida) was born on 25 Apr 1954 in Boston, MA. David married Gloria Ruth BLITSTEIN on 17 Aug 1981 in Oceanside, NY. Gloria was born on 16 Sep 1956 in Brooklyn, NY. They had the following children:

27 Benjamin Douglas SOLOMON was born on 17 Oct 1984 in Washington, DC.

28 Michael Alan SOLOMON was born on 1 Mar 1987 in Washington, DC.

13. James Mark RADNER (Babette SOLOMON, Maida) was born on 30 Aug 1955 in Boston, MA. James married Mary Paul (Polly) WELLS on 20 Jun 1993 in Philadelphia, PA. Mary was born on 17 Oct 1953 in San Juan, Puerto Rico. They had the following children:

29 George Henry RADNER was born on 22 Dec 1995 in Washington, DC.

30 Claire Paul RADNER was born on 16 May 2000 in Washington, DC.

15. Wendy Herman RADNER (Babette SOLOMON, Maida) was born on 7 May 1957 in Boston, MA. Wendy married Kenneth James TAUBES on 21 Jun 1981 in Belmont, MA. Kenneth was born on 26 Apr 1958. They had the following children:

31 Marcy Lynn TAUBES was born on 27 Jun 1985.

32 Valerie Michelle TAUBES was born on 19 May 1988.

33 Evan Seth TAUBES was born on 27 Feb 1991.

16. Madeline Andrea SOLOMON (H. Eric SOLOMON, Maida) was born on 9 May 1960 in Columbus, OH. She had the following child:

34 Naomi Song SOLOMON was born on 25 Sep 1981 in San Francisco, CA.

17. William Daniel SOLOMON (H. Eric SOLOMON, Maida) was born on 13 Mar 1964 in Baltimore, MD. William married Molly Suzanne HUTTON on 15 May 1999. Molly was born on 11 Jan 1966. They had the following child:

35 Eliott H. SOLOMON was born in Mar 2001 in California.

Maida and Harry's great-grandchild

20. Keisha SANCHEZ (Maida Elizabeth SOLOMON, Peter Herman SOLOMON, Maida) was born on 10 May 1975 in San Salvador. She had the following child:

36 Dequan Akeem SANCHEZ was born on 30 Dec 1993 in Boston, MA.

References

Written or stated quotes by Maida Herman Solomon in the preceding text derive from these sources:

The Arthur E. and Elizabeth Schlesinger Library; Radcliffe Institute, Harvard University, Cambridge, MA.

The Colonel Miriam E. Perry Goll Archives; Simmons College, Boston, MA, Smith College, Northampton, MA.

The William E. Weiner Oral History Library; American Jewish Committee, New York, NY.

Also:

Dorfman, Rachelle A., MSS, (ed.), *Paradigms of Clinical Social Work*, Brunner/Mazel Publishers, New York, NY, 1988.

Edward, Joyce, and Sanville, Jean (eds.), *Fostering Healing and Growth, A Psychoanalytic Social Work Approach*, Jason Aronson, Inc., Northvale, NJ, 1996.

Encyclopedia of Social Work, 16th Edition, National Association of Social Workers, 1971.

Greenblatt, M., Albert R. Moore, and M. Solomon, *The Prevention of Hospitalization*, Grune and Stratton, Inc., New York, NY, 1963.

Greenblatt, M., M.H. Solomon, A.S. Evans, and G. Brooks, *Drugs and Social Therapies in Chronic Schizophrenia*, Charles Thomas, Springfield, IL, 1965.

Herrera, E., E. Dawson, and M. Solomon, *A History of America's First Urban Mental Health Residence*, Rutland Corner House, 1978.

Hyman, Paula E., and Deborah Dash More (ed.), *Jewish Women in America: An Historical Encyclopedia*, Vol. 2, Routledge, NY, 1997, p. 1287.

Kerber, Linda K., *Toward an Intellectual History of Women*, The University of North Carolina Press, Chapel Hill, NC, 1997.

Lunbeck, Elizabeth, *The Psychiatric Persuasion: Knowledge, Gender and Power in Modern America*, Princeton University Press, Princeton, NJ, 1994.

Reinherz, H.Z., "College Student Volunteers as Case Aides in a State Hospital for Children," *The American Journal for Orthopsychiatry*, 33, 1964, p. 544. *Report of the First Seventy-five Years of the Simmons College School of Social Work*, Simmons College, Boston, MA, 1979.

Schneider, Dorothy, and Carl J. Schneider, *American Women in the Progressive Era: 1900-1920*, Doubleday, New York, NY, 1979.

Solomon, Barbara Miller, *Pioneers in Service: A History of the Associated Jewish Philanthropies of Boston*, 1956.

————, *In the Company of Educated Women: A History of Women and Higher Education in America*, Yale University Press, New York, NY, 1985.

Solomon, Harry C., and Maida H. Solomon, *Syphilis of the Innocent*, Social Hygiene Board, Washington, DC, 1920.

Umbarger, C.C., J.S. Dalismer, A.P. Morrison, and P.R. Bregin, *College Students in a Mental Hospital*, Grune & Stratton, New York, NY, 1962.

Wilensky, Harold L., and Lebeaux, Charles N, *Industrial Society and Social Welfare*, Russell Sage Foundation, New York, NY, 1958.

Selected Publications of Maida Herman Solomon

Davis, Philip and Maida Herman (eds.), *Field of Social Work,* Small, Maynard & Co., Boston, MA, 1915.

Solomon, Harry, C., and Maida H. Solomon, "The Family Neurosyphilitic," *Mental Hygiene*, April, 1918.

————, *Syphilis of the Innocent*, Social Hygiene Board, Washington, DC, 1920.

Solomon, Maida H., "Psychiatric Social Work," *Smith Alumni Quarterly*, January, 1920.

Solomon, Harry, C. and Maida H. Solomon, "Effects of Syphilis on the Families of Syphilitics Seen in the Late Stages," *Social Hygiene Quarterly*, October, 1920.

————, "The Social Worker's Approach to the Family of the Syphilitic," *Hospital Social Service*, June, 1921.

Solomon, Harry C., and Maida H. Solomon, "A Study of the Economic Status of 41 Paretic Patients and Their Families," *Mental Hygiene*, July 1921.

Evans, Anne S., Dexter M. Bullard, Jr., and Maida H. Solomon, "The Family as a Potential Resource in the Rehabilitation of the Chronic Schizophrenic Patient: A Study of 60 Patients," *American Journal of Psychiatry*, 117:12, June 1961, p. 1075-1083.

Deykin, Eva, Shirley Jacobson, and Maida H. Solomon, *Clinical and Metabolic Studies of Depressive Illness*: "The PSW Recording Instrument: A Guide for Use of Measuring Scales for Monthly Relative Observation," December, 1962.

Greenblatt, Milton, Robert F. Moore, Robert S. Albert, and Maida H. Solomon, *Prevention of Hospitalization*, Grune & Stratton, Inc., New York, 1963.

Greenblatt, Milton, Maida H. Solomon, Anne S. Evans, and George Brooks, *Drugs and Social Therapies in Chronic Schizophrenia*, Charles C. Thomas Publisher, Springfield, IL, 1965.

Hartman, Ernest, Betty Ann Glasser, Milton Greenblatt, Maida H. Solomon, and Daniel Levenson, *Adolescents in a Mental Hospital*, Grune & Stratton, 1968.

Herrera, Elizabeth G., Betty Glasser Lifson, Ernest Hartman, and Maida H. Solomon, "A 10 Year Follow-up of 55 Hospitalized Adolescents," *American Psychiatric Association*, 1974.

Herrera, Elizabeth, Emma Dawson, and Maida H. Solomon, *A History of America's First Urban Mental Health Residence*, Rutland Corner House, June 1978.

Lifson, Betty, Joan Martin, and Maida H. Solomon, *A Story of Innovation at Boston State Hospital* (Vista Program), 1978-1979.

Selected Publications of
Anne S. Evans, MSW

Goldberg, Margaret F., Anne S. Evans and Katharine Cole, "Associate Leaders—The Utilization and Training of Volunteers in a Psychiatric Social Work Setting," *British Journal of Social Work*, Vol. 3,1: May 1973, p. 55-63.

Evans, Anne S. and Dexter Bullard, Jr., "The Family as a Potential Resource in the Rehabilitation of the Chronic Schizophrenic Patient: A Study of Twenty-four Patients," *Mental Hygiene*, Vol. 44, No. 1, January 1960, p. 64-73.

Evans, Anne S., *The Relationship of Drugs and Milieu in the Treatment of Chronic Schizophrenia*, published in VA-NIMH Transactions of the Fifth Research Conference of Cooperative Chemotherapy Studies in Psychiatry and Research Approaches to Mental Illness, Vol. V, Veterans Administration, Washington, DC, December 1960, p. 140-146.

Evans, Anne, S., Dexter Bullard, Jr., and Maida H. Solomon, "The Family as a Potential Resource in the Rehabilitation of the Chronic Schizophrenic Patient: A Study of 60 Patients and Their Families," *American Journal of Psychiatry*, Vol. 117, No. 12, June 1961, p. 1075-1083.

Evans, Anne S., and Margaret Wessler, "The Research-Oriented Single Home Follow-up Interview: Its Validity and Effectiveness as a Methodological Tool," *Journal of Health and Human Behavior*, Fall 1963, Vol. 4, p. 214-217.

Evans, Anne S., and Maida H. Solomon, "Family Attitudes Toward and Interactions with Chronic Schizophrenic Patients: A Three Year Follow-up Study," presented at Group-Without-A-Name Conference, Vermont, 1963.

Gelineau, Victor, and Anne S. Evans, "Volunteer Case Aides Rehabilitate Chronic Patients," *Hospital and Community Psychiatry*, March 1970, p. 90-93.

Greenblatt, Milton, Maida H. Solomon, Anne S. Evans and George Brooks (eds.), *Drugs and Social Therapies in Chronic Schizophrenia*, Charles C. Thomas Publisher, Springfield, IL, 1965.

Evans, Anne S., and Margaret Goldberg, "Catholic Seminarians in a Secular Institution," *Mental Hygiene*, Vol. 54, No. 4, October 1970, p. 559-564.

Evans, Anne S., *The Case Aide Program at the Boston State Hospital—Its Structure and Development*, presented at the Massachusetts Association for Mental Health Conference, February 29, 1972.

Maguire, Robert E., and Anne S. Evans, "Interdisciplinary Supervision: A Dynamic Model for Growth and Integration Skills," *Camillian,* Vol. XII, No. 4, November 1974.

Evans, Anne S., "The Volunteer Case Aide Program: An Adventure in Community Outreach," *Volunteer Administration*, Association of Voluntary Action Scholars, Vol. VIII, 3-4, 1975.

Acknowledgments

Thanks are due to several children and grandchildren of Maida Herman Solomon: in particular to Joe, son, and his wife, Carolyn, for their advice and encouragement and for photographs of Maida and Harry at their 60th anniversary celebration and a photograph of his grandparents Joseph and Hennie Herman; to Eric, son, who offered his recollections of his parents; and to David Solomon, grandson of Maida, who researched and documented the Solomon family tree and the Herman genealogy. Barbara Miller Solomon, late daughter-in-law, and Maida E. Solomon, grandchild, contributed good advice to the project.

So too, the author's appreciation is extended to the Arthur and Elizabeth Schlesinger Library, Radcliffe Institute, Harvard University, Cambridge, MA. Marie-Helene Gold, photography coordinator at the Schlesinger, has been particularly helpful.

Claire Goodwin, archivist of the Colonel Miriam E. Perry Goll Archives, Simmons College, Boston, was very helpful in obtaining pictures of 51 Commonwealth Avenue (home of the Simmons College School of Social Work from 1945 to 2002). Also, thanks to the William E. Weiner Oral History Collection of the American Jewish Committee; New York and Smith College collections. Each contributed important source materials.

Thanks too are due to several of Maida's former students/colleagues and friends of the author, whose interesting and substantive comments have been included: Mary Breslin, MSW; Eva Y. Deykin, PhD; Margaret F. Goldberg, MSW; Mollie C. Grob, MSW; Elizabeth Gould Herrera, MSW; Betty Ann Glasser Lifson, MSW; Joan P. Morse, MSW; and Shirley Jacobson, MSW.

Katharine Cole, MSW, helped to edit several early sections of the work. Mary Breslin, MSW, reviewed many photographs and identified classmates.

Readers included the late Milton Greenblatt, MD, Director of Research at Massachusetts Mental Health Center, Superintendent of Boston State Hospital, Commissioner of Mental Health, MA; Joan Pinanski Morse, MSW; Carolyn Thomas, PhD; Diana Waldfogel, MSW, former Dean, Simmons Graduate School of Social Work; Fr. George Winchester, SJ; and Robert E. and Sally Wyner.

Special thanks go to Professor Emeritus Carolyn Thomas, who encouraged me to rework and publish the manuscript. I received the benefit of her wisdom as former director of the doctoral program at the Boston College School of Social Work.

I am grateful to Miles F. Shore, MD, for his personal and insightful perspective of Maida; to Nona Rooney for her remarkable artistic talent; to Ed Sugarman for his remarkable photographic talent as evidenced by a picture of the author; to George Trask, publisher, Coastal Villages Press; to Sally Sisson, proofreader; and to Jennifer Fox, typist extraordinaire.

I also thank those who read the manuscript in its various stages, made suggestions, and wrote reviews: Mary Breslin, MSW; Don Lipsitt, MD; Golnar Simpson, DSW; and Carolyn Thomas, PhD.

And a special word of love and gratitude to my husband, Sam, who whole-heartedly supported my interest in having Maida's story published. John and Julie, our son and daughter-in-law, and daughter Laura (Maida Herman Solomon's godchild) and son-in-law Lee, have been there with their words of encouragement. I am truly blessed.

About the Author
Anne S. Evans

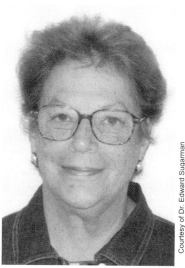

Anne S. Evans graduated from the Simmons College School of Social Work, Boston, MA (1957). She met Mrs. Solomon in the latter's capacity as Professor of Social Economy and Director of the psychiatric social work sequence at the school. Upon her mandatory retirement from the college (1957), Maida H. Solomon became the author's first research supervisor at the Psycho. Mrs. Evans was employed as a research psychiatric social worker in an NIMH- funded project on "Drugs and Social Therapy in Chronic Schizophrenia." The results of that study were published in 1965 by Charles C. Thomas, edited by Greenblatt, Solomon (MH), Evans, and Brooks.

In 1963, Mrs. Evans' work took her to the Boston State Hospital where she helped to develop, implement, and supervise volunteers and staff, as well as direct research activities in a study utilizing college students and community-based volunteers in the treatment of long-time hospitalized patients. Maida H. Solomon continued to work with the psychiatric social work staff in both a supervisory and consultative capacity.

In both research assignments, Mrs. Evans was author and/or co-author of a number of research reports and journal articles. One such collaborative paper with Margaret Goldberg and Katharine Cole received the Maida H. Solomon Award (Simmons College School of Social Work) in 1972. This work was later translated and published in German.

Mrs. Evans was one of several "Maida's Girls" (later renamed "The Maida H. Solomon Research Associates"). This began as a group of several psychiatric social work researchers (later including colleagues and family members) whose purpose was to celebrate her birthday, her work, and her commitment to psychiatric social work and community psychiatry.

The author was an incorporator and charter member of The Massachusetts Academy of Psychiatric Social Work, now known as The Massachusetts Society of Clinical Social Work, and served as its third president from 1979 until 1983.

From 1980 to 1996, Mrs. Evans engaged in a private practice in Newton, MA. She now resides in South Carolina. She is the wife of Samuel N. Evans; mother of two, John R. Evans of Briarcliff Manor, NY, and Laura J. Stone of Cohasset, MA; and grandmother of five.

Biographical Sketch of
Miles F. Shore, MD

Miles F. Shore, MD, is Bullard Professor of Psychiatry, Harvard Medical School and Visiting Scholar at the John F. Kennedy School of Government, Harvard University. He has bachelor's degrees from the University of Chicago and Harvard College, and received his MD from Harvard Medical School. Dr. Shore interned at the University of Illinois Research and Education Hospitals, was a psychiatric resident at the Massachusetts Mental Health Center and at Beth Israel Hospital in Boston, and graduated form the Boston Psychoanalytic Institute.

Dr. Shore began his psychiatric teaching career at Harvard and in 1964 became Director of both Community Psychiatry and the Mental Health Center at Tufts University School of Medicine. He was appointed Professor of Psychiatry at Tufts in 1971 and, a year later, Associate Dean for Community Affairs and Director for Community Health and Ambulatory Care at the New England Medical Center Hospital. In 1975 he moved to Harvard as Bullard Professor of Psychiatry and served as Superintendent of the Massachusetts Mental Health Center from then until June 30, 1993.

Dr. Shore has been a consultant to a wide variety of community agencies, clinics, and hospitals, including the Tufts-Delta Health Center in Mound Bayou, Mississippi; the World Council of Churches; the U. S. Department of Health and Human Services Task Force on Homeless and Severe Mental Illness; the American Managed Behavioral Healthcare Association (AMBHA); the Midwest Healthcare Marketing Association (MHMA); Community Behavioral Care in Philadelphia; and Merit Behavioral Care. As consultant to AMBHA, he organized and participated in the development of the first two iterations of a collection of tools for investigations of permutation groups (PERMS), the AMBHA instrument for documenting quality, a number of whose items have been incorporated in the most recent Health Plan Employer Data and Information Set (HEDIS) test set.

From 1985 to 1992 he was director of the Program for Chronic Mental Illness of the Robert Wood Johnson Foundation. He has served as a member of the Board of Directors of the Massachusetts Hospital Association, the Medical Foundation in Boston, and as Chair of the Governing Council on Mental Health and Substance Abuse Services of the American Hospital Association. During 1996-1997 he was president of the American College of Psychiatrists. He is co-director, with Joseph P. Newhouse, PhD, of an executive program in health policy for physicians and health care leaders, titled "Understanding the New World of Health Care."

Awards and honors include the Annual Award for Administrative Psychiatry of the American Psychiatric Association in 1987; the National Alliance for the Mentally Ill Exemplary Psychiatrist Award in 1992; the 1993 Bowis Award for service to the American College of Psychiatry; and the Distinguished Service Award from the Department of Mental Health, Commonwealth of Massachusetts in 1993.

Colophon

Tabby Manse

Coastal Villages Press is dedicated to helping
to preserve the timeless values of traditional
places along America's Atlantic coast—
building houses to endure through
the centuries; living in harmony
with the natural environment;
honoring history, culture,
family and friends—
and helping to
make
these
values
relevant
today.
This
book
was
completed on
July 20, 2003, at Stonington, Maine.
It was designed and set by George Graham Trask
in Bembo, a typeface inspired by the Italian renaissance.